Teen Health Series

Fitness Information For Teens, Fourth Edition

Fitness Information For Teens,
Fourth Edition

Health Tips About Exercise And Active Lifestyles

Including Facts About Healthy Muscles And Bones,
Starting And Maintaining Fitness Plans, Aerobic Fitness,
Stretching And Strength Training, Sports Safety, And
Suggestions For Team Athletes And Individuals

OMNIGRAPHICS
615 Griswold, Ste. 901
Detroit, MI 48226

OMNIGRAPHICS
Siva Ganesh Maharaja, *Managing Editor*

* * *

Copyright © 2018 Omnigraphics
ISBN 978-0-7808-1585-8
E-ISBN 978-0-7808-1586-5

Library of Congress Cataloging-in-Publication Data

Names: Omnigraphics, Inc., issuing body.

Title: Fitness information for teens: health tips about exercise and active lifestyles including facts about healthy muscles and bones, starting and maintaining fitness plans, aerobic fitness, stretching and strength training, sports safety, and suggestions for team athletes and individuals.

Description: Fourth edition. | Detroit,MI: Omnigraphics, [2018] | Series: Teen health series | Audience: Grade 9 to 12. | Includes bibliographical references and index.

Identifiers: LCCN 2017034133 (print) | LCCN 2017036003 (ebook) | ISBN 9780780815865 (eBook) | ISBN 9780780815858 (hardcover: alk. paper)

Subjects: LCSH: Physical fitness for youth.

Classification: LCC RJ133 (ebook) | LCC RJ133.F58 2018 (print) | DDC 613.7/043--dc23

LC record available at https://lccn.loc.gov/2017034133

Table Of Contents

Part Three: Exercise Fundamentals

Part Four: Activities For Team Athletes And Individuals

Part Five: Sports Safety

Part Six: Overcoming Obstacles To Fitness

Part Seven: Health And Wellness Trends

Part Eight: If You Need More Information

Preface

About This Book

When teens adopt healthy and active habits, the rewards can persist for a lifetime. According to the Centers for Disease Control and Prevention (CDC), the numerous benefits of physical fitness include weight control, stronger bones and muscles, and improved mental health and mood. In addition, by avoiding inactivity teens can help reduce the risks that cardiovascular disease, metabolic syndrome, type 2 diabetes, and some types of cancer will develop later in their lives.

Despite the benefits, however, many young people fail to meet guidelines for physical activity. A study from the CDC reported that less than 3 in 10 (27.1%) of high school students participate in at least 60 minutes per day of physical activity on all 7 days of the week. Furthermore, only 21.6% of 6 to 19-year-old children and adolescents in the Unites States attained 60 or more minutes of moderate-to-vigorous physical activity on at least 5 days per week.

Fitness Information For Teens, Fourth Edition offers teens a comprehensive, fact-based guide for living a healthy and active lifestyle. The book includes information about the developing body, the components of fitness, and making and maintaining a fitness plan. It discusses exercise fundamentals and activities for team athletes and individuals—whether beginners or experienced competitors. Sports safety concerns, nutrition challenges, and suggestions for overcoming obstacles concerning fitness and change are also addressed. The book concludes with information about the President's Challenge and directories of additional resources.

How To Use This Book

This book is divided into parts and chapters. Parts focus on broad areas of interest; chapters are devoted to single topics within a part.

Part One: Your Body And The Components Of Fitness begins with a definition of fitness, and it goes on to explain the importance of developing muscular strength, endurance, and flexibility. Additional chapters discuss other components of mental and physical fitness, including proper nutrition, weight management, and sleep requirements.

Part Two: Making And Maintaining A Fitness Plan provides guidance for taking the first steps on the path toward fitness and continuing on toward reachable goals. It offers suggestions for evaluating current fitness levels, identifying targets for improvement, and making progress toward the development of a physically active lifestyle.

Part Three: Exercise Fundamentals describes the basic categories of exercises, including aerobic exercise, muscle-strengthening exercise, bone-strengthening exercise, and exercises that help promote flexibility and balance. It also discusses how to measure exercise intensity, and it includes examples of various types of activities and their intensity levels.

Part Four: Activities For Team Athletes And Individuals provides facts about a wide range of team sports and individual activities that can be part of a well-rounded fitness program.

Part Five: Sports Safety discusses practical tips for preventing injuries. It reminds readers who participate in physical activities about the importance of following safety guidelines, including warming up and cooling down, using protective equipment such as helmets and appropriate footwear, taking precautions in adverse weather conditions, and avoiding dehydration.

Part Six: Overcoming Obstacles To Fitness describes the challenge of staying on course to meet fitness goals and offers suggestions for maintaining motivation. It explains commonly encountered barriers to fitness, including sports injuries and pre-existing conditions such as asthma, diabetes, or physical disabilities. It also discusses problems associated with compulsive exercise, female athlete triad, and the dangers of using steroids or other performance-enhancing substances.

Part Seven: Health and Wellness Trends discusses recent developments in health and fitness including online training, wellness tourism, and wearable technology.

Part Eight: If You Need More Information explains how the President's Challenge can help people set and reach fitness goals, and it offers directories of general fitness organizations and resources for more information about specific sports and activities.

Bibliographic Note

This volume contains documents and excerpts from publications issued by the following government agencies: Air Force Public Affairs Agency (AFPAA); Centers for Disease Control and Prevention (CDC); Federal Communications Commission (FCC); Federal Trade Commission (FTC); *Go4Life*; National Aeronautics and Space Administration (NASA); National Center for Biotechnology Information (NCBI); National Center for Complementary and Integrative Health (NCCIH); National Heart, Lung, and Blood Institute (NHLBI); National Institute of Arthritis and Musculoskeletal and Skin Diseases (NIAMS); National Institute of Diabetes and Digestive and Kidney Diseases (NIDDK); National Institute on

Drug Abuse (NIDA); National Institute on Drug Abuse (NIDA) for Teens; National Institutes of Health (NIH); National Interagency Fire Center (NIFC); National Oceanic and Atmospheric Administration (NOAA); Office of Dietary Supplements (ODS); Office of Disease Prevention and Health Promotion (ODPHP); Office on Women's Health (OWH); President's Council on Fitness, Sports & Nutrition (PCFSN); Small Business Administration (SBA); U.S. Consumer Product Safety Commission (CPSC); U.S. Customs and Border Protection (CBP); U.S. Department of Agriculture (USDA); U.S. Department of Health and Human Services (HHS); U.S. Department of Veterans Affairs (VA); U.S. Environmental Protection Agency (EPA); U.S. Food and Drug Administration (FDA); and U.S. Public Health Service Commissioned Corps (PHSCC).

It may also contain original material produced by Omnigraphics and reviewed by medical consultants.

The photograph on the front cover is © Clique Images/Unsplash.

Medical Review

Omnigraphics contracts with a team of qualified, senior medical professionals who serve as medical consultants for the *Teen Health Series*. As necessary, medical consultants review reprinted and originally written material for currency and accuracy. Citations including the phrase, Reviewed (month, year)" indicate material reviewed by this team. Medical consultation services are provided to the *Teen Health Series* editors by:

Dr. Vijayalakshmi, MBBS, DGO, MD
Dr. Senthil Selvan, MBBS, DCH, MD
Dr. K. Sivanandham, MBBS, DCH, MS (Research), PhD

About The *Teen Health Series*

At the request of librarians serving today's young adults, the *Teen Health Series* was developed as a specially focused set of volumes within Omnigraphics' *Health Reference Series*. Each volume deals comprehensively with a topic selected according to the needs and interests of people in middle school and high school. Teens seeking preventive guidance, information about disease warning signs, medical statistics, and risk factors for health problems will find answers to their questions in the *Teen Health Series*. The *Series*, however, is not intended to serve as a tool for diagnosing illness, in prescribing treatments, or as a substitute for the physician/patient relationship. All people concerned about medical symptoms or the possibility of disease are encouraged to seek professional care from an appropriate healthcare provider.

If there is a topic you would like to see addressed in a future volume of the *Teen Health Series*, please write to:

Editor
Teen Health Series
Omnigraphics
615 Griswold, Ste. 901
Detroit, MI 48226

A Note About Spelling And Style

Teen Health Series editors use *Stedman's Medical Dictionary* as an authority for questions related to the spelling of medical terms and the *Chicago Manual of Style* for questions related to grammatical structures, punctuation, and other editorial concerns. Consistent adherence is not always possible, however, because the individual volumes within the *Series* include many documents from a wide variety of different producers and copyright holders, and the editor's primary goal is to present material from each source as accurately as is possible following the terms specified by each document's producer. This sometimes means that information in different chapters may follow other guidelines and alternate spelling authorities. For example, occasionally a copyright holder may require that eponymous terms be shown in possessive forms (Crohn's disease vs. Crohn disease) or that British spelling norms be retained (leukaemia vs. leukemia).

Part One
Your Body And The Components Of Fitness

Chapter 1

What Is Fitness?

Defining Fitness

Physical fitness is to the human body what fine tuning is to an engine. It enables us to perform up to our potential. Fitness can be described as a condition that helps us look, feel, and do our best. More specifically, it is: "The ability to perform daily tasks vigorously and alertly, with energy left over for enjoying leisure-time activities and meeting emergency demands. It is the ability to endure, to bear up, to withstand stress, to carry on in circumstances where an unfit person could not continue, and is a major basis for good health and well-being." Physical fitness involves the performance of the heart and lungs, and the muscles of the body. And, since what we do with our bodies also affects what we can do with our minds, fitness influences to some degree qualities such as mental alertness and emotional stability.

As you undertake your fitness program, it's important to remember that fitness is an individual quality that varies from person to person. It is influenced by age, sex, heredity, personal habits, exercise, and eating practices. You can't do anything about the first three factors. However, it is within your power to change and improve the others where needed.

About This Chapter: This chapter includes text excerpted from "Fitness Fundamentals: Guidelines For Personal Exercise Programs," President's Council on Fitness, Sports, & Nutrition (PCFSN), 2011. Reviewed September 2017.

Knowing The Basics

Physical fitness is most easily understood by examining its components, or "parts." There is widespread agreement that these four components are basic:

- **Cardiorespiratory Endurance**—the ability to deliver oxygen and nutrients to tissues, and to remove wastes, over sustained periods of time. Long runs and swims are among the methods employed in measuring this component.

- **Muscular Strength**—the ability of a muscle to exert force for a brief period of time. Upper-body strength, for example, can be measured by various weightlifting exercises.

- **Muscular Endurance**—the ability of a muscle, or a group of muscles, to sustain repeated contractions or to continue applying force against a fixed object. Pushups are often used to test endurance of arm and shoulder muscles.

- **Flexibility**—the ability to move joints and use muscles through their full range of motion. The sit-and-reach test is a good measure of flexibility of the lower back and backs of the upper legs.

- **Body Composition** is often considered a component of fitness. It refers to the makeup of the body in terms of lean mass (muscle, bone, vital tissue, and organs) and fat mass. An optimal ratio of fat to lean mass is an indication of fitness, and the right types of exercises will help you decrease body fat and increase or maintain muscle mass.

A Workout Schedule

How often, how long and how hard you exercise, and what kinds of exercises you do should be determined by what you are trying to accomplish. Your goals, your present fitness level, age, health, skills, interest, and convenience are among the factors you should consider. For example, an athlete training for high-level competition would follow a different program than a person whose goals are good health and the ability to meet work and recreational needs.

Your exercise program should include something from each of the four basic fitness components described previously. Each workout should begin with a warm-up and end with a cooldown. As a general rule, space your workouts throughout the week and avoid consecutive days of hard exercise.

Here are the amounts of activity necessary for the average healthy person to maintain a minimum level of overall fitness. Included are some of the popular exercises for each category.

- **Warm-up:** Five to 10 minutes of exercise such as walking, slow jogging, knee lifts, arm circles, or trunk rotations. Low intensity movements that simulate movements to be used in the activity can also be included in the warm-up.

- **Muscular strength:** A minimum of two 20-minute sessions per week that include exercises for all the major muscle groups. Lifting weights is the most effective way to increase strength.

- **Muscular endurance:** At least three 30-minute sessions each week that include exercises such as calisthenics, pushups, situps, pullups, and weight training for all the major muscle groups.

- **Cardiorespiratory endurance:** At least three 20-minute bouts of continuous aerobic (activity requiring oxygen) rhythmic exercise each week. Popular aerobic conditioning activities include brisk walking, jogging, swimming, cycling, rope-jumping, rowing, cross-country skiing, and some continuous action games like racquetball and handball.

- **Flexibility:** 10–12 minutes of daily stretching exercises performed slowly, without a bouncing motion. This can be included after a warm-up or during a cooldown.

- **Cool down:** A minimum of 5–10 minutes of slow walking, low-level exercise, combined with stretching.

A Matter Of Principle

The keys to selecting the right kinds of exercises for developing and maintaining each of the basic components of fitness are found in these principles:

- **Specificity:** Pick the right kind of activities to affect each component. Strength training results in specific strength changes. Also, train for the specific activity you're interested in. For example, optimal swimming performance is best achieved when the muscles involved in swimming are trained for the movements required. It does not necessarily follow that a good runner is a good swimmer.

- **Overload:** Work hard enough, at levels that are vigorous and long enough to overload your body above its resting level, to bring about improvement.

- **Regularity:** You can't hoard physical fitness. At least three balanced workouts a week are necessary to maintain a desirable level of fitness.

- **Progression:** Increase the intensity, frequency and/or duration of activity over periods of time in order to improve.

Some activities can be used to fulfill more than one of your basic exercise requirements. For example, in addition to increasing cardiorespiratory endurance, running builds muscular endurance in the legs, and swimming develops the arm, shoulder and chest muscles. If you select the proper activities, it is possible to fit parts of your muscular endurance workout into your cardiorespiratory workout and save time.

---

10 Tips To Healthy Eating And Physical Activity For You

1. Start your day with breakfast.

2. Get Moving!

3. Snack smart.

4. Work up a sweat.

5. Balance your food choices--don't eat too much of any one thing.

6. Get fit with friends or family.

7. Eat more grains, fruits, and vegetables.

8. Join in physical activities at school.

9. Foods aren't good or bad.

10. Make healthy eating and physical activities fun!

Measuring Your Heart Rate

Heart rate is widely accepted as a good method for measuring intensity during running, swimming, cycling, and other aerobic activities. Exercise that doesn't raise your heart rate to a certain level and keep it there for 20 minutes won't contribute significantly to cardiovascular fitness.

The heart rate you should maintain is called your target heart rate. There are several ways of arriving at this figure. One of the simplest is: maximum heart rate (220 - age) x 70 percent. Thus, the target heart rate for a 40 year-old would be 126.

Some methods for figuring the target rate take individual differences into consideration. Here is one of them:

• Subtract age from 220 to find maximum heart rate.

• Subtract resting heart rate (see below) from maximum heart rate to determine heart rate reserve.

- Take 70 percent of heart rate reserve to determine heart rate raise.
- Add heart rate raise to resting heart rate to find target rate.

Resting heart rate should be determined by taking your pulse after sitting quietly for five minutes. When checking heart rate during a workout, take your pulse within five seconds after interrupting exercise because it starts to go down once you stop moving. Count pulse for 10 seconds and multiply by six to get the per-minute rate.

Controlling Your Weight

The key to weight control is keeping energy intake (food) and energy output (physical activity) in balance. When you consume only as many calories as your body needs, your weight will usually remain constant. If you take in more calories than your body needs, you will put on excess fat. If you expend more energy than you take in you will burn excess fat. Exercise plays an important role in weight control by increasing energy output, calling on stored calories for extra fuel. Studies show that not only does exercise increase metabolism during a workout, but it causes your metabolism to stay increased for a period of time after exercising, allowing you to burn more calories.

How much exercise is needed to make a difference in your weight depends on the amount and type of activity, and on how much you eat. Aerobic exercise burns body fat. A medium-sized adult would have to walk more than 30 miles to burn up 3,500 calories, the equivalent of one pound of fat. Although that may seem like a lot, you don't have to walk the 30 miles all at once. Walking a mile a day for 30 days will achieve the same result, providing you don't increase your food intake to negate the effects of walking.

If you consume 100 calories a day more than your body needs, you will gain approximately 10 pounds in a year. You could take that weight off, or keep it off, by doing 30 minutes of moderate exercise daily. The combination of exercise and diet offers the most flexible and effective approach to weight control. Since muscle tissue weighs more than fat tissue, and exercise develops muscle to a certain degree, your bathroom scale won't necessarily tell you whether or not you are "fat." Well muscled individuals, with relatively little body fat, invariably are "overweight" according to standard weight charts. If you are doing a regular program of strength training, your muscles will increase in weight, and possibly your overall weight will increase. Body composition is a better indicator of your condition than body weight.

Lack of physical activity causes muscles to get soft, and if food intake is not decreased, added body weight is almost always fat. Once-active people, who continue to eat as they always have after settling into sedentary lifestyles, tend to suffer from "creeping obesity."

Chapter 2

Physical Activity And Its Importance

What Is Physical Activity?

Physical activity simply means movement of the body that uses energy. Walking, gardening, briskly pushing a baby stroller, climbing the stairs, playing soccer, or dancing the night away are all good examples of being active. For health benefits, physical activity should be moderate or vigorous intensity.

Moderate physical activities include:

- Walking briskly (about 3½ miles per hour)

- Bicycling (less than 10 miles per hour)

- General gardening (raking, trimming shrubs)

- Dancing

- Golf (walking and carrying clubs)

- Water aerobics

- Canoeing

- Tennis (doubles)

About This Chapter: Text beginning with the heading "What Is Physical Activity?" is excerpted from "Physical Activity," ChooseMyPlate.gov, U.S. Department of Agriculture (USDA), June 10, 2015; Text under the heading "What Being Active Does For Your Body" is excerpted from "Why Physical Activity Is Important," girlshealth.gov, Office on Women's Health (OWH), March 27, 2015.

Vigorous physical activities include:

- Running/jogging (5 miles per hour)

- Walking very fast (4½ miles per hour)

- Bicycling (more than 10 miles per hour)

- Heavy yard work, such as chopping wood

- Swimming (freestyle laps)

- Aerobics

- Basketball (competitive)

- Tennis (singles)

You can choose moderate or vigorous intensity activities, or a mix of both each week. Activities can be considered vigorous, moderate, or light in intensity. This depends on the extent to which they make you breathe harder and your heart beat faster.

Only moderate and vigorous intensity activities count toward meeting your physical activity needs. With vigorous activities, you get similar health benefits in half the time it takes you with moderate ones. You can replace some or all of your moderate activity with vigorous activity. Although you are moving, light intensity activities do not increase your heart rate, so you should not count these towards meeting the physical activity recommendations. These activities include walking at a casual pace, such as while grocery shopping, and doing light household chores.

Why Is Physical Activity Important?

Regular physical activity can produce long-term health benefits. People of all ages, shapes, sizes, and abilities can benefit from being physically active. The more physical activity you do, the greater the health benefits.

Being physically active can help you:

- Increase your chances of living longer

- Feel better about yourself

- Decrease your chances of becoming depressed

- Sleep well at night

- Move around more easily

- Have stronger muscles and bones

- Stay at or get to a healthy weight

- Be with friends or meet new people

- Enjoy yourself and have fun

When you are not physically active, you are more likely to:

- Get heart disease

- Get type 2 diabetes

- Have high blood pressure

- Have high blood cholesterol

- Have a stroke

Physical activity and nutrition work together for better health. Being active increases the amount of calories burned. As people age their metabolism slows, so maintaining energy balance requires moving more and eating less.

Some types of physical activity are especially beneficial:

- **Aerobic activities** make you breathe harder and make your heart beat faster. Aerobic activities can be moderate or vigorous in their intensity. Vigorous activities take more effort than moderate ones. For moderate activities, you can talk while you do them, but you can't sing. For vigorous activities, you can only say a few words without stopping to catch your breath.

- **Muscle strengthening activities** make your muscles stronger. These include activities like push-ups and lifting weights. It is important to work all the different parts of the body your legs, hips, back, chest, stomach, shoulders, and arms.

- **Bone strengthening activities** make your bones stronger. Bone strengthening activities, like jumping, are especially important for children and adolescents. These activities produce a force on the bones that promotes bone growth and strength.

- **Balance and stretching activities** enhance physical stability and flexibility, which reduces risk of injuries. Examples are gentle stretching, dancing, yoga, martial arts, and tai chi.

How Much Physical Activity Is Needed?

Physical activity is important for everyone, but how much you need depends on your age.

Children And Adolescents (6–17 Years)

Children and adolescents should do 60 minutes or more of physical activity each day. Most of the 60 minutes should be either moderate- or vigorous-intensity aerobic physical activity, and should include vigorous intensity physical activity at least 3 days a week. As part of their 60 or more minutes of daily physical activity, children and adolescents should include muscle strengthening activities, like climbing, at least 3 days a week and bone strengthening activities, like jumping, at least 3 days a week. Children and adolescents are often active in short bursts of time rather than for sustained periods of time, and these short bursts can add up to meet physical activity needs. Physical activities for children and adolescents should be developmentally appropriate, fun, and offer variety.

Physical activity is generally safe for everyone. The health benefits you gain from being active are far greater than the chances of getting hurt. Here are some things you can do to stay safe while you are active:

- If you haven't been active in a while, start slowly and build up.

- Learn about the types and amounts of activity that are right for you.

- Choose activities that are appropriate for your fitness level.

- Build up the time you spend before switching to activities that take more effort.

- Use the right safety gear and sports equipment.

- Choose a safe place to do your activity.

- See a healthcare provider if you have a health problem.

How Many Calories Does Physical Activity Burn?

A 154-pound man who is 5'10" will use up (burn) about the number of calories listed doing each activity below. Those who weigh more will use more calories; those who weigh less will use fewer calories. The calorie values listed include both calories used by the activity and the calories used for normal body functioning during the activity time.

Table 2.1. Physical Activity Calorie Chart

Approximate Calories Used (Burned) By A 154-Pound Man		
MODERATE physical activities:	In 1 hour	In 30 minutes
Hiking	370	185
Light gardening/yard work	330	165
Dancing	330	165

Table 2.1. Continued

Approximate Calories Used (Burned) By A 154-Pound Man		
MODERATE physical activities:	**In 1 hour**	**In 30 minutes**
Golf (walking and carrying clubs)	330	165
Bicycling (less than 10 mph)	290	145
Walking (3.5 mph)	280	140
Weight training (general light workout)	220	110
Stretching	180	90
VIGOROUS physical activities:	**In 1 hour**	**In 30 minutes**
Running/jogging (5 mph)	590	295
Bicycling (more than 10 mph)	590	295
Swimming (slow freestyle laps)	510	255
Aerobics	480	240
Walking (4.5 mph)	460	230
Heavy yard work (chopping wood)	440	220
Weight lifting (vigorous effort)	440	220
Basketball (vigorous)	440	220

Tips For Increasing Physical Activity
Make Physical Activity A Regular Part Of The Day

Choose activities that you enjoy and can do regularly. Fitting activity into a daily routine can be easy—such as taking a brisk 10 minute walk to and from the parking lot, bus stop, or subway station. Or, join an exercise class. Keep it interesting by trying something different on alternate days. Every little bit adds up and doing something is better than doing nothing.

Make sure to do at least 10 minutes of activity at a time, shorter bursts of activity will not have the same health benefits. For example, walking the dog for 10 minutes before and after work or adding a 10 minute walk at lunchtime can add to your weekly goal. Mix it up. Swim, take a yoga class, garden, or lift weights. To be ready anytime, keep some comfortable clothes and a pair of walking or running shoes in the car and at the office.

More Ways To Increase Physical Activity

At home:

- Join a walking group in the neighborhood or at the local shopping mall. Recruit a partner for support and encouragement.

- Push the baby in a stroller.

- Get the whole family involved—enjoy an afternoon bike ride with your kids.

- Walk up and down the soccer or softball field sidelines while watching the kids play.

- Walk the dog—don't just watch the dog walk.

- Clean the house or wash the car.

- Walk, skate, or cycle more, and drive less.

- Do stretches, exercises, or pedal a stationary bike while watching television.

- Mow the lawn with a push mower.

- Plant and care for a vegetable or flower garden.

- Play with the kids—tumble in the leaves, build a snowman, splash in a puddle, or dance to favorite music.

- Exercise to a workout video.

At work:

- Get off the bus or subway one stop early and walk or skate the rest of the way.

- Replace a coffee break with a brisk 10-minute walk. Ask a friend to go with you.

- Take part in an exercise program at work or a nearby gym.

- Join the office softball team or walking group.

At play:

- Walk, jog, skate, or cycle.

- Swim or do water aerobics.

- Take a class in martial arts, dance, or yoga.

- Golf (pull cart or carry clubs).

- Canoe, row, or kayak.

- Play racquetball, tennis, or squash.

- Ski cross-country or downhill.

- Play basketball, softball, or soccer.

- Hand cycle or play wheelchair sports.

- Take a nature walk.

- Most important—have fun while being active!

What Being Active Does For Your Body

Being physically active is great for your muscles, heart, and lungs. Some other possible benefits of activity include:

- **Building strong bones.** Your body creates the most bone when you are a kid and a teen. You can learn more about how to build great bones.

- **Promoting a healthy weight.** Obesity is a serious problem among kids in the United States. It can lead to problems with your sleep, knees, heart, emotions, and more, but exercise can help.

- **Helping avoid diabetes.** A lot more young people are getting diabetes than ever before. Regular physical activity can help prevent one type of diabetes.

- **Building healthy habits.** If you get used to being active now, you will more likely keep it up when you're older. You'll thank yourself later!

- **Fighting cancer.** Research shows that exercise may help protect against certain kinds of cancer, including breast cancer.

- **Helping prevent high blood pressure.** The number of kids with high blood pressure is growing. High blood pressure makes your heart and arteries work extra hard to pump blood. It also puts you at risk for things like kidney and eye disease.

Are you worried that exercise will bulk you up? Exercising won't give you big, bulging muscles. It takes a very intense weightlifting program to get a bodybuilder look. And exercise and other forms of physical activity can help if you need to lose weight or want to stay a healthy weight.

Chapter 3

Meeting Your Muscles

Basic Facts About Muscles

Did you know you have more than 600 muscles in your body? These muscles help you move, lift things, pump blood through your body, and even help you breathe.

When you think about your muscles, you probably think most about the ones you can control. These are your voluntary muscles, which means you can control their movements. They are also called skeletal muscles, because they attach to your bones and work together with your bones to help you walk, run, pick up things, play an instrument, throw a baseball, kick a soccer ball, push a lawnmower, or ride a bicycle. The muscles of your mouth and throat even help you talk!

Keeping your muscles healthy will help you to be able to walk, run, jump, lift things, play sports, and do all the other things you love to do. Exercising, getting enough rest, and eating a balanced diet will help to keep your muscles healthy for life.

Why Healthy Muscles Matter To You

Healthy muscles let you move freely and keep your body strong. They help you to enjoy playing sports, dancing, walking the dog, swimming, and other fun activities. And they help you do those other (not so fun) things that you have to do, like making the bed, vacuuming the carpet, or mowing the lawn.

Strong muscles also help to keep your joints in good shape. If the muscles around your knee, for example, get weak, you may be more likely to injure that knee. Strong muscles also help you keep your balance, so you are less likely to slip or fall.

About This Chapter: This chapter includes text excerpted from "Healthy Muscles Matter," National Institute of Arthritis and Musculoskeletal and Skin Diseases (NIAMS), October 15, 2015.

And remember—the activities that make your skeletal muscles strong will also help to keep your heart muscle strong!

Different Kinds Of Muscles Have Different Jobs

Skeletal muscles are connected to your bones by tough cords of tissue called tendons. As the muscle contracts, it pulls on the tendon, which moves the bone. Bones are connected to other bones by ligaments, which are like tendons and help hold your skeleton together.

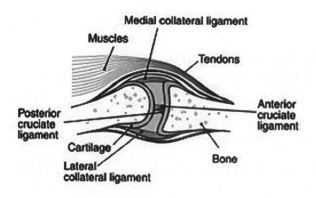

Figure 3.1. A Joint Showing Muscles, Ligaments, And Tendons

Smooth muscles are also called involuntary muscles since you have no control over them. Smooth muscles work in your digestive system to move food along and push waste out of your body. They also help keep your eyes focused without your having to think about it.

Cardiac muscle. Did you know your heart is also a muscle? It is a specialized type of involuntary muscle. It pumps blood through your body, changing its speed to keep up with the demands you put on it. It pumps more slowly when you're sitting or lying down, and faster when you're running or playing sports and your skeletal muscles need more blood to help them do their work.

Most skeletal muscles have names that describe some feature of the muscle. Often several criteria are combined into one name. Associating the muscle's characteristics with its name will help you learn and remember them. The following are some terms relating to muscle features that are used in naming muscles.

- **Size:** vastus (huge); maximus (large); longus (long); minimus (small); brevis (short).

- **Shape:** deltoid (triangular); rhomboid (like a rhombus with equal and parallel sides); latissimus (wide); teres (round); trapezius (like a trapezoid, a four-sided figure with two sides parallel).

- **Direction of fibers:** rectus (straight); transverse (across); oblique (diagonally); orbicularis (circular).

- **Location:** pectoralis (chest); gluteus (buttock or rump); brachii (arm); supra- (above); infra- (below); sub- (under or beneath); lateralis (lateral).

- **Number of origins:** biceps (two heads); triceps (three heads); quadriceps (four heads).

- **Origin and insertion:** sternocleidomastoideus (origin on the sternum and clavicle, insertion on the mastoid process); brachioradialis (origin on the brachium or arm, insertion on the radius).

- **Action:** abductor (to abduct a structure); adductor (to adduct a structure); flexor (to flex a structure); extensor (to extend a structure); levator (to lift or elevate a structure); masseter (a chewer).

(Source: "Muscle Groups," National Cancer Institute (NCI).)

Physical Activity

When you make your muscles work by being physically active, they respond by growing stronger. They may even get bigger by adding more muscle tissue. This is how bodybuilders get such big muscles, but your muscles can be healthy without getting that big.

There are lots of activities you can do for your muscles. Walking, jogging, lifting weights, playing tennis, climbing stairs, jumping, and dancing are all good ways to exercise your muscles. Swimming and biking will also give your muscles a good workout. It's important to get different kinds of activities to work all your muscles. And any activity that makes you breathe harder and faster will help exercise that important heart muscle as well!

Get 60 minutes of physical activity every day. It doesn't have to be all at once, but it does need to be in at least 10-minute increments to count toward your 60 minutes of physical activity per day.

Eat A Healthy Diet

You really don't need a special diet to keep your muscles in good health. Eating a balanced diet will help manage your weight and provide a variety of nutrients for your muscles and overall health. A balanced diet:

- Emphasizes fruits, vegetables, whole grains, and fat-free or low-fat dairy products like milk, cheese, and yogurt.

- Includes protein from lean meats, poultry, seafood, beans, eggs, and nuts.

- Is low in solid fats, saturated fats, cholesterol, salt (sodium), added sugars, and refined grains.

- Is as low as possible in *trans* fats.

- Balances calories taken in through food with calories burned in physical activity to help maintain a healthy weight.

As you grow and become an adult, iron is an important nutrient, especially for girls. Not getting enough iron can cause anemia which can make you feel weak and tired because your muscles don't get enough oxygen. This can also keep you from getting enough activity to keep your muscles healthy. You can get iron from foods like lean beef, chicken and turkey; beans and peas; spinach; and iron-enriched breads and cereals. You can also get iron from dietary supplements, but it's always good to check with a doctor first.

Some people think that supplements will make their muscles bigger and stronger. However, supplements like creatine can cause serious side effects, and protein and amino acid supplements are no better than getting protein from your food. Using steroids to increase your muscles is illegal (unless a doctor has prescribed them for a medical problem), and can have dangerous side effects. No muscle-building supplement can take the place of good nutrition and proper training.

Prevent Injuries

To help prevent sprains, strains, and other muscle injuries:

- **Warm up and cool down.** Before exercising or playing sports, warm-up exercises, such as stretching and light jogging, may make it less likely that you'll strain a muscle. They are called warm-up exercises because they make the muscles warmer—and more flexible. Cool-down exercises loosen muscles that have tightened during exercise.

- **Wear the proper protective gear** for your sport, for example pads or helmets. This will help reduce your risk for injuring your muscles or joints.

- Remember to **drink lots of water** while you're playing or exercising, especially in warm weather. If your body's water level gets too low (dehydration),you could get dizzy or even pass out. Dehydration can cause many medical problems.

- **Don't try to "play through the pain."** If something starts to hurt, STOP exercising or playing. You might need to see a doctor, or you might just need to rest the injured part for a while.

- If you have been inactive, **"start low and go slow"** by gradually increasing how often and how long activities are done. Increase physical activity gradually over time.

- **Be careful when you lift heavy objects.** Keep your back straight and bend your knees to lift the object. This will protect the muscles in your back and put most of the weight on the strong muscles in your legs. Get someone to help you lift something heavy.

Start Now

Keeping your muscles healthy will help you have more fun and enjoy the things you do. Healthy muscles will help you look your best and feel full of energy. Start good habits now, while you are young, and you'll have a better chance of keeping your muscles healthy for the rest of your life.

Chapter 4

Bone Health

Why Does Bone Health Matter?

Our bones support us and allow us to move. They protect our brain, heart, and other organs from injury. Our bones also store minerals such as calcium and phosphorous, which help keep our bones strong, and release them into the body when we need them for other uses.

There are many things we can do to keep our bones healthy and strong. Eating foods rich in calcium and vitamin D, getting plenty of exercise, and having good health habits help keep our bones healthy.

But if we don't eat right and don't get enough of the right kinds of exercise, our bones can become weak and even break. Broken bones (called fractures) can be painful and sometimes need surgery to heal. They can also cause long-lasting health problems.

What Can I Do To Make My Bones Healthier?

It is never too early or too late to take care of your bones. The following steps can help you improve your bone health:

- **Eat a well-balanced diet rich in calcium and vitamin D.** Good sources of calcium include low-fat dairy products, and foods and drinks with added calcium. Good sources of vitamin D include egg yolks, saltwater fish, liver, and milk with vitamin D. Some

---

About This Chapter: Text beginning with the heading "Why Does Bone Health Matter?" is excerpted from "Bone Health For Life: Health Information Basics For You And Your Family," National Institute of Arthritis and Musculoskeletal and Skin Diseases (NIAMS), July 2014. Reviewed September 2017; Text beginning with the heading "Why Exercise?" is excerpted from "Exercise For Your Bone Health," National Institute of Arthritis and Musculoskeletal and Skin Diseases (NIAMS), May 2015.

people may need to take nutritional supplements in order to get enough calcium and vitamin D. The charts below show how much calcium and vitamin D you need each day. Fruits and vegetables also contribute other nutrients that are important for bone health.

- **Get plenty of physical activity.** Like muscles, bones become stronger with exercise. The best exercises for healthy bones are strength-building and weight-bearing, like walking, climbing stairs, lifting weights, and dancing. Try to get 30 minutes of exercise each day.

- **Live a healthy lifestyle.** Don't smoke, and, if you choose to drink alcohol, don't drink too much.

- **Talk to your doctor about your bone health.** Go over your risk factors with your doctor and ask if you should get a bone density test. If you need it, your doctor can order medicine to help prevent bone loss and reduce your chances of breaking a bone.

- **Prevent falls.** Falling down can cause a bone to break, especially in someone with osteoporosis. But most falls can be prevented. Check your home for dangers like loose rugs and poor lighting. Have your vision checked. Increase your balance and strength by walking every day and taking classes like tai chi, yoga, or dancing.

Sources Of Calcium

- Tofu (calcium fortified)
- Soy milk (calcium fortified)
- Green leafy vegetables (e.g., broccoli, brussels sprouts, mustard greens, kale)
- Chinese cabbage or bok choy
- Beans/legumes
- Tortillas
- Sardines/salmon with edible bones
- Shrimp
- Orange juice (calcium fortified)
- Pizza
- Bread
- Nuts/almonds
- Dairy products (e.g., milk, cheese, yogurt)

Table 4.1. Nutrition Table

Recommended Calcium And Vitamin D Intakes		
Life-Stage Group	**Calcium mg/day**	**Vitamin D (IU/day)**
Infants 0 to 6 months	200	400
Infants 6 to 12 months	260	400
1 to 3 years old	700	600
4 to 8 years old	1,000	600
9 to 13 years old	1,300	600
14 to 18 years old	1,300	600
19 to 30 years old	1,000	600
31 to 50 years old	1,000	600
51- to 70-year-old males	1,000	600
51- to 70-year-old females	1,200	600
>70 years old	1,200	800
14 to 18 years old, pregnant/lactating	1,300	600
19 to 50 years old, pregnant/lactating	1,000	600
Definitions: mg = milligrams; IU = International Units		

(Source: Food And Nutrition Board (FNB), Institute of Medicine (IOM), National Academy of Sciences (NAS).)

Why Exercise?

Like muscle, bone is living tissue that responds to exercise by becoming stronger. Young women and men who exercise regularly generally achieve greater peak bone mass (maximum bone density and strength) than those who do not. For most people, bone mass peaks during the third decade of life. After that time, we can begin to lose bone. Women and men older than age 20 can help prevent bone loss with regular exercise. Exercising allows us to maintain muscle strength, coordination, and balance, which in turn helps to prevent falls and related fractures. This is especially important for older adults and people who have been diagnosed with osteoporosis.

The Best Bone-Building Exercise

The best exercise for your bones is the weight-bearing kind, which forces you to work against gravity. Some examples of weight-bearing exercises include weight training, walking, hiking, jogging, climbing stairs, tennis, and dancing. Examples of exercises that are not weight-bearing include swimming and bicycling. Although these activities help build and maintain strong muscles and have excellent cardiovascular benefits, they are not the best way to exercise your bones.

Exercise Tips

If you have health problems—such as heart trouble, high blood pressure, diabetes, or obesity, check with your doctor before you begin a regular exercise program. According to the Surgeon General, the optimal goal is at least 30 minutes of physical activity on most days, preferably daily. Listen to your body.

When starting an exercise routine, you may have some muscle soreness and discomfort at the beginning, but this should not be painful or last more than 48 hours. If it does, you may be working too hard and need to ease up. Stop exercising if you have any chest pain or discomfort, and see your doctor before your next exercise session. If you have osteoporosis, ask your doctor which activities are safe for you. If you have low bone mass, experts recommend that you protect your spine by avoiding exercises or activities that flex, bend, or twist it.

Furthermore, you should avoid high impact exercise to lower the risk of breaking a bone. You also might want to consult with an exercise specialist to learn the proper progression of activity, how to stretch and strengthen muscles safely, and how to correct poor posture habits. An exercise specialist should have a degree in exercise physiology, physical education, physical therapy, or a similar specialty. Be sure to ask if he or she is familiar with the special needs of people with osteoporosis.

A Complete Osteoporosis Program

Remember, exercise is only one part of an osteoporosis prevention or treatment program. Like a diet rich in calcium and vitamin D, exercise helps strengthen bones at any age. But proper exercise and diet may not be enough to stop bone loss caused by medical conditions, menopause, or lifestyle choices such as tobacco use and excessive alcohol consumption. It is important to speak with your doctor about your bone health. Discuss whether you might be a candidate for a bone mineral density test. If you are diagnosed with low bone mass, ask what medications might help keep your bones strong.

Chapter 5

Your Heart And Lungs

What Is The Heart?

Your heart is a muscular organ that pumps blood to your body. Your heart is at the center of your circulatory system. This system consists of a network of blood vessels, such as arteries, veins, and capillaries. These blood vessels carry blood to and from all areas of your body. An electrical system controls your heart and uses electrical signals to contract the heart's walls. When the walls contract, blood is pumped into your circulatory system. Inlet and outlet valves in your heart chambers ensure that blood flows in the right direction.

Your heart is vital to your health and nearly everything that goes on in your body. Without the heart's pumping action, blood can't move throughout your body. Your blood carries the oxygen and nutrients that your organs need to work well. Blood also carries carbon dioxide (a waste product) to your lungs so you can breathe it out.

A healthy heart supplies your body with the right amount of blood at the rate needed to work well. If disease or injury weakens your heart, your body's organs won't receive enough blood to work normally.

Anatomy Of The Heart

Your heart is located under your ribcage in the center of your chest between your right and left lungs. Its muscular walls beat, or contract, pumping blood to all parts of your body. The size

About This Chapter: Text under the heading "What Is The Heart?" is excerpted from "How The Heart Works," National Heart, Lung, and Blood Institute (NHLBI), November 17, 2011. Reviewed September 2017; Text under the heading "What Are The Lungs?" is excerpted from "How The Lungs Work," National Heart, Lung, and Blood Institute (NHLBI), July 17, 2012. Reviewed September 2017.

of your heart can vary depending on your age, size, and the condition of your heart. A normal, healthy, adult heart usually is the size of an average clenched adult fist. Some diseases can cause the heart to enlarge.

The Exterior Of The Heart

The heart has four chambers:

- The heart's upper chambers, the right and left atria.

- The heart's lower chambers, the right and left ventricles.

Some of the main blood vessels (arteries and veins) that make up your circulatory system are directly connected to the heart.

The Right Side Of Your Heart

The superior and inferior vena cavae are the largest veins in your body. After your body's organs and tissues have used the oxygen in your blood, the vena cavae carry the oxygen-poor blood back to the right atrium of your heart. The superior vena cava carries oxygen-poor blood from the upper parts of your body, including your head, chest, arms, and neck. The inferior vena cava carries oxygen-poor blood from the lower parts of your body.

The oxygen-poor blood from the vena cavae flows into your heart's right atrium and then to the right ventricle. From the right ventricle, the blood is pumped through the pulmonary

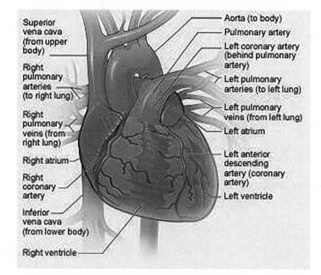

Figure 5.1. Front Surface Of The Heart

arteries to your lungs. The oxygen-rich blood passes from your lungs back to your heart through the pulmonary veins.

The Left Side Of Your Heart

Oxygen-rich blood from your lungs passes through the pulmonary veins. The blood enters the left atrium and is pumped into the left ventricle. From the left ventricle, the oxygen-rich blood is pumped to the rest of your body through the aorta. The aorta is the main artery that carries oxygen-rich blood to your body. Like all of your organs, your heart needs oxygen-rich blood. As blood is pumped out of your heart's left ventricle, some of it flows into the coronary arteries. Your coronary arteries are located on your heart's surface at the beginning of the aorta. They carry oxygen-rich blood to all parts of your heart.

The Interior Of The Heart

Heart Chambers

Heart is divided into four chambers. The two upper chambers of your heart are called the atria. They receive and collect blood. The two lower chambers of your heart are called ventricles. The ventricles pump blood out of your heart to other parts of your body.

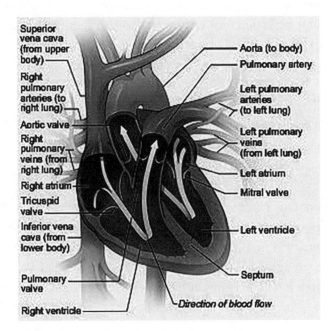

Figure 5.2. Cross-Section Of The Heart

The Septum

An internal wall of tissue divides the right and left sides of your heart. This wall is called the septum. The area of the septum that divides the atria is called the atrial or interatrial septum. The area of the septum that divides the ventricles is called the ventricular or interventricular septum.

Heart Valves

Heart's four valves include the aortic valve, the tricuspid valve, the pulmonary valve, and the mitral valve.

Blood Flow

Blood enters the right atrium of your heart from the superior and inferior vena cavae. From the right atrium, blood is pumped into the right ventricle. From the right ventricle, blood is pumped to your lungs through the pulmonary arteries. Oxygen-rich blood coming from your lungs through the pulmonary veins into your heart's left atrium. From the left atrium, the blood is pumped into the left ventricle. The left ventricle pumps the blood to the rest of your body through the aorta.

For the heart to work well, your blood must flow in only one direction. Your heart's valves make this possible. Both of your heart's ventricles have an "in" (inlet) valve from the atria and an "out" (outlet) valve leading to your arteries. Healthy valves open and close in exact coordination with the pumping action of your heart's atria and ventricles. Each valve has a set of flaps called leaflets or cusps that seal or open the valve. This allows blood to pass through the chambers and into your arteries without backing up or flowing backward.

Circulation And Blood Vessels

Your heart and blood vessels make up your overall blood circulatory system. Your blood circulatory system is made up of four subsystems.

Arterial Circulation

Arterial circulation is the part of your circulatory system that involves arteries, like the aorta and pulmonary arteries. Arteries are blood vessels that carry blood away from your heart. (The exception is the coronary arteries, which supply your heart muscle with oxygen-rich blood.) Healthy arteries are strong and elastic (stretchy). They become narrow between heartbeats, and they help keep your blood pressure consistent. This helps blood move through your body.

Arteries branch into smaller blood vessels called arterioles. Arteries and arterioles have strong, flexible walls that allow them to adjust the amount and rate of blood flowing to parts of your body.

Venous Circulation

Venous circulation is the part of your circulatory system that involves veins, like the vena cavae and pulmonary veins. Veins are blood vessels that carry blood to your heart. Veins have thinner walls than arteries. Veins can widen as the amount of blood passing through them increases.

Capillary Circulation

Capillary circulation is the part of your circulatory system where oxygen, nutrients, and waste pass between your blood and parts of your body. Capillaries are very small blood vessels. They connect the arterial and venous circulatory subsystems.

The importance of capillaries lies in their very thin walls. Oxygen and nutrients in your blood can pass through the walls of the capillaries to the parts of your body that need them to work normally. Capillaries' thin walls also allow waste products like carbon dioxide to pass from your body's organs and tissues into the blood, where it's taken away to your lungs.

Pulmonary Circulation

Pulmonary circulation is the movement of blood from the heart to the lungs and back to the heart again. Pulmonary circulation includes both arterial and venous circulation. Oxygen-poor blood is pumped to the lungs from the heart (arterial circulation). Oxygen-rich blood moves from the lungs to the heart through the pulmonary veins (venous circulation).

Pulmonary circulation also includes capillary circulation. Oxygen you breathe in from the air passes through your lungs into your blood through the many capillaries in the lungs. Oxygen-rich blood moves through your pulmonary veins to the left side of your heart and out of the aorta to the rest of your body. Capillaries in the lungs also remove carbon dioxide from your blood so that your lungs can breathe the carbon dioxide out into the air.

Your Heart's Electrical System

Your heart's electrical system controls all the events that occur when your heart pumps blood. The electrical system also is called the cardiac conduction system. If you've ever seen the heart test called an EKG (electrocardiogram), you've seen a graphical picture of the heart's electrical activity.

Your heart's electrical system is made up of three main parts:

• The sinoatrial (SA) node, located in the right atrium of your heart

- The atrioventricular (AV) node, located on the interatrial septum close to the tricuspid valve

- The His-Purkinje system, located along the walls of your heart's ventricles

A heartbeat is a complex series of events. These events take place inside and around your heart. A heartbeat is a single cycle in which your heart's chambers relax and contract to pump blood. This cycle includes the opening and closing of the inlet and outlet valves of the right and left ventricles of your heart. Each heartbeat has two basic parts: diastole and systole. During diastole, the atria and ventricles of your heart relax and begin to fill with blood.

At the end of diastole, your heart's atria contract (atrial systole) and pump blood into the ventricles. The atria then begin to relax. Your heart's ventricles then contract (ventricular systole), pumping blood out of your heart.

Each beat of your heart is set in motion by an electrical signal from within your heart muscle. In a normal, healthy heart, each beat begins with a signal from the SA node. This is why the SA node sometimes is called your heart's natural pacemaker. Your pulse, or heart rate, is the number of signals the SA node produces per minute. The signal is generated as the vena cavae fill your heart's right atrium with blood from other parts of your body. The signal spreads across the cells of your heart's right and left atria. This signal causes the atria to contract. This action pushes blood through the open valves from the atria into both ventricles.

The signal arrives at the AV node near the ventricles. It slows for an instant to allow your heart's right and left ventricles to fill with blood. The signal is released and moves along a pathway called the bundle of His, which is located in the walls of your heart's ventricles. From the bundle of His, the signal fibers divide into left and right bundle branches through the Purkinje fibers. These fibers connect directly to the cells in the walls of your heart's left and right ventricles. The signal spreads across the cells of your ventricle walls, and both ventricles contract. However, this doesn't happen at exactly the same moment.

The left ventricle contracts an instant before the right ventricle. This pushes blood through the pulmonary valve (for the right ventricle) to your lungs, and through the aortic valve (for the left ventricle) to the rest of your body. As the signal passes, the walls of the ventricles relax and await the next signal. This process continues over and over as the atria refill with blood and more electrical signals come from the SA node.

Heart Disease

Your heart is made up of many parts working together to pump blood. In a healthy heart, all the parts work well so that your heart pumps blood normally. As a result, all parts of your body that depend on the heart to deliver blood also stay healthy. Heart disease can disrupt a heart's normal electrical system and pumping functions. Diseases and conditions of the heart's muscle make it hard for your heart to properly pump blood. Damaged or diseased blood vessels make the heart work harder than normal. Problems with the heart's electrical system, called arrhythmias can make it hard for the heart to pump blood efficiently.

Three Moves For Health

While not usually aerobic, the activities below offer numerous health benefits and are enjoyable ways to get and stay in shape. All are offered at many YMCAs, community or recreation centers, and gyms.

- **Yoga** is a system of physical postures, stretching, and breathing techniques that can improve flexibility, balance, muscle strength, and relaxation. Many styles are available, ranging from slow and gentle to athletic and vigorous. A study found that regular yoga practice may help to minimize weight gain in middle age.

- **Tai chi** is an ancient Chinese practice based on shifting body weight through a series of slow movements that flow rhythmically together into one graceful gesture. This gentle, calming practice can help to improve flexibility and balance, and it gradually builds muscle strength.

- **Pilates** is a body conditioning routine that seeks to strengthen the body's "core" (torso), usually through a series of mat exercises. Another Pilates method uses special exercise machines, available at some health clubs. The practice can strengthen and tone muscles as well as increase flexibility.

(Source: "Your Guide To Physical Activity And Your Heart," National Heart, Lung, and Blood Institute (NHLBI).)

What Are The Lungs?

Your lungs are organs in your chest that allow your body to take in oxygen from the air. They also help remove carbon dioxide (a waste gas that can be toxic) from your body. The lungs' intake of oxygen and removal of carbon dioxide is called gas exchange. Gas exchange is part of breathing. Breathing is a vital function of life; it helps your body work properly. Other organs and tissues also help make breathing possible.

Endurance, or aerobic, activities increase your breathing and heart rate. They keep your heart, lungs, and circulatory system healthy and improve your overall fitness. Building your endurance makes it easier to carry out many of your everyday activities.

- Brisk walking or jogging
- Yard work (mowing, raking, digging)
- Dancing

(Source: "4 Types Of Exercise," Go4Life, National Institutes of Health (NIH).)

The Respiratory System

The respiratory system is made up of organs and tissues that help you breathe. The main parts of this system are the airways, the lungs and linked blood vessels, and the muscles that enable breathing.

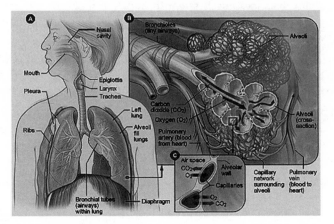

Figure 5.3. Respiratory System

Figure A shows the location of the respiratory structures in the body. Figure B is an enlarged view of the airways, alveoli (air sacs), and capillaries (tiny blood vessels). Figure C is a closeup view of gas exchange between the capillaries and alveoli. CO_2 is carbon dioxide, and O_2 is oxygen.

Airways

The airways are pipes that carry oxygen-rich air to your lungs. They also carry carbon dioxide, a waste gas, out of your lungs. The airways include your:

- Nose and linked air passages (called nasal cavities)
- Mouth
- Larynx, or voice box

- Trachea, or windpipe

- Tubes called bronchial tubes or bronchi, and their branches

Air first enters your body through your nose or mouth, which wets and warms the air. (Cold, dry air can irritate your lungs). The air then travels through your voice box and down your windpipe. The windpipe splits into two bronchial tubes that enter your lungs. A thin flap of tissue called the epiglottis covers your windpipe when you swallow.

This prevents food and drink from entering the air passages that lead to your lungs. Except for the mouth and some parts of the nose, all of the airways have special hairs called cilia that are coated with sticky mucus. The cilia trap germs and other foreign particles that enter your airways when you breathe in air. These fine hairs then sweep the particles up to the nose or mouth. From there, they're swallowed, coughed, or sneezed out of the body. Nose hairs and mouth saliva also trap particles and germs.

Lungs And Blood Vessels

Your lungs and linked blood vessels deliver oxygen to your body and remove carbon dioxide from your body. Your lungs lie on either side of your breastbone and fill the inside of your chest cavity. Your left lung is slightly smaller than your right lung to allow room for your heart.

Within the lungs, your bronchi branch into thousands of smaller, thinner tubes called bronchioles. These tubes end in bunches of tiny round air sacs called alveoli. Each of these air sacs is covered in a mesh of tiny blood vessels called capillaries. The capillaries connect to a network of arteries and veins that move blood through your body.

The pulmonary artery and its branches deliver blood rich in carbon dioxide (and lacking in oxygen) to the capillaries that surround the air sacs. Inside the air sacs, carbon dioxide moves from the blood into the air. At the same time, oxygen moves from the air into the blood in the capillaries. The oxygen-rich blood then travels to the heart through the pulmonary vein and its branches. The heart pumps the oxygen-rich blood out to the body.

The lungs are divided into five main sections called lobes. Some people need to have a diseased lung lobe removed. However, they can still breathe well using the rest of their lung lobes.

Muscles Used For Breathing

Muscles near the lungs help expand and contract (tighten) the lungs to allow breathing. These muscles include:

- Diaphragm

- Intercostal muscles

- Abdominal muscles

- Muscles in the neck and collarbone area

The diaphragm is a dome-shaped muscle located below your lungs. It separates the chest cavity from the abdominal cavity. The diaphragm is the main muscle used for breathing. The intercostal muscles are located between your ribs. They also play a major role in helping you breathe. Beneath your diaphragm are abdominal muscles. They help you breathe out when you're breathing fast (for example, during physical activity). Muscles in your neck and collarbone area help you breathe in when other muscles involved in breathing don't work well, or when lung disease impairs your breathing.

What Happens When You Breathe?

Breathing In (Inhalation)

When you breathe in, or inhale, your diaphragm contracts (tightens) and moves downward. This increases the space in your chest cavity, into which your lungs expand. The intercostal muscles between your ribs also help enlarge the chest cavity. They contract to pull your rib cage both upward and outward when you inhale.

As your lungs expand, air is sucked in through your nose or mouth. The air travels down your windpipe and into your lungs. After passing through your bronchial tubes, the air finally reaches and enters the alveoli (air sacs).

Through the very thin walls of the alveoli, oxygen from the air passes to the surrounding capillaries (blood vessels). A red blood cell protein called hemoglobin helps move oxygen from the air sacs to the blood. At the same time, carbon dioxide moves from the capillaries into the air sacs. The gas has traveled in the bloodstream from the right side of the heart through the pulmonary artery.

Oxygen-rich blood from the lungs is carried through a network of capillaries to the pulmonary vein. This vein delivers the oxygen-rich blood to the left side of the heart. The left side of the heart pumps the blood to the rest of the body. There, the oxygen in the blood moves from blood vessels into surrounding tissues.

Breathing Out (Exhalation)

When you breathe out, or exhale, your diaphragm relaxes and moves upward into the chest cavity. The intercostal muscles between the ribs also relax to reduce the space in the chest cavity. As the space in the chest cavity gets smaller, air rich in carbon dioxide is forced out of your lungs and windpipe, and then out of your nose or mouth.

Breathing out requires no effort from your body unless you have a lung disease or are doing physical activity. When you're physically active, your abdominal muscles contract and push your diaphragm against your lungs even more than usual. This rapidly pushes air out of your lungs.

What Controls Your Breathing?

A respiratory control center at the base of your brain controls your breathing. This center sends ongoing signals down your spine and to the muscles involved in breathing. These signals ensure your breathing muscles contract (tighten) and relax regularly. This allows your breathing to happen automatically, without you being aware of it.

To a limited degree, you can change your breathing rate, such as by breathing faster or holding your breath. Your emotions also can change your breathing. For example, being scared or angry can affect your breathing pattern.

Your breathing will change depending on how active you are and the condition of the air around you. For example, you need to breathe more often when you do physical activity. In contrast, your body needs to restrict how much air you breathe if the air contains irritants or toxins.

To adjust your breathing to changing needs, your body has many sensors in your brain, blood vessels, muscles, and lungs. Sensors in the brain and in two major blood vessels detect carbon dioxide or oxygen levels in your blood and change your breathing rate as needed.

Sensors in the airways detect lung irritants. The sensors can trigger sneezing or coughing. In people who have asthma, the sensors may cause the muscles around the airways in the lungs to contract. This makes the airways smaller. Sensors in the alveoli (air sacs) can detect fluid buildup in the lung tissues. These sensors are thought to trigger rapid, shallow breathing. Sensors in your joints and muscles detect movement of your arms or legs. These sensors may play a role in increasing your breathing rate when you're physically active.

Lung Diseases And Conditions

Breathing is a complex process. If injury, disease, or other factors affect any part of the process, you may have trouble breathing. For example, the fine hairs (cilia) that line your upper airways may not trap all of the germs you breathe in. These germs can cause an infection in your bronchial tubes (bronchitis) or deep in your lungs (pneumonia). These infections cause a buildup of mucus or fluid that narrows the airways and limits airflow in and out of your lungs.

If you have asthma, breathing in certain substances that you're sensitive to can trigger your airways to narrow. This makes it hard for air to flow in and out of your lungs. Over a long period, breathing in cigarette smoke or air pollutants can damage the airways and air sacs. This can lead to a disease called COPD (chronic obstructive pulmonary disease). COPD prevents proper airflow in and out of your lungs and can hinder gas exchange in the air sacs.

An important step to breathing is the movement of your diaphragm and other muscles in your chest, neck, and abdomen. This movement lets you inhale and exhale. Nerves that run from your brain to these muscles control their movement. Damage to these nerves in your upper spinal cord can cause breathing to stop, unless a machine is used to help you breathe. (This machine is called a ventilator or a respirator.)

A steady flow of blood in the small blood vessels that surround your air sacs is vital for gas exchange. Long periods of inactivity or surgery can cause a blood clot called a pulmonary embolism (PE) to block a lung artery. A PE can reduce or block the flow of blood in the small blood vessels and hinder gas exchange.

Chapter 6

Teen Nutrition

Eat Smart And Be Active As You Grow: Ten Healthy Tips For Teen Girls

Young girls, ages 10 to 19, have a lot of changes going on in their bodies. Building healthier habits will help you—now as a growing teen—and later in life. Growing up means you are in charge of foods you eat and the time you spend being physically active every day.

1. Build Strong Bones

A good diet and regular physical activity can build strong bones throughout your life. Choose fat-free or low-fat milk, cheeses, and yogurt to get the vitamin D and calcium your growing bones need. Strengthen your bones three times a week doing activities such as running, gymnastics, and skating.

2. Cut Back On Sweets

Cut back on sugary drinks. Many 12-ounce cans of soda have 10 teaspoons of sugar in them. Drink water when you are thirsty. Sipping water and cutting back on cakes, candies, and sweets helps to maintain a healthy weight.

About This Chapter: Text under the heading "Eat Smart And Be Active As You Grow: Ten Healthy Tips For Teen Girls" is excerpted from "Eat Smart And Be Active As You Grow," ChooseMyPlate.gov, U.S. Department of Agriculture (USDA), January 2014. Reviewed September 2017; Text under the heading "Choose The Foods You Need To Grow: Ten Tips For Teen Guys" is excerpted from "10 Tips: Choose The Foods You Need To Grow," ChooseMyPlate.gov, U.S. Department of Agriculture (USDA), August 4, 2017.

3. Power Up With Whole Grain

Fuel your body with nutrient-packed whole-grain foods. Make sure that at least half your grain foods are whole grains such as brown rice, whole-wheat breads, and popcorn.

4. Choose Vegetables Rich In Color

Brighten your plate with vegetables that are red, orange or dark green. Try acorn squash, cherry tomatoes or sweet potatoes. Spinach and beans also provide vitamins like folate and minerals like potassium that are essential for healthy growth.

5. Check Nutrition Facts Labels For Iron

Read Nutrition Facts labels to find foods containing iron. Most protein foods like meat, poultry, eggs, and beans have iron, and so do fortified breakfast cereals and breads.

Nutrition Facts Label

The Nutrition Facts Label can help you learn about the nutrient content of many foods in your diet.

It also enables you to compare foods to make healthy choices.

The Nutrition Facts Label must list: Total fat, saturated fat, trans fat, cholesterol, sodium, total carbohydrate, dietary fiber, sugars, protein, vitamin A, vitamin C, calcium, and iron.

The Nutrition Facts Label may also list: Monounsaturated fat, polyunsaturated fat, soluble fiber, insoluble fiber, sugar alcohol, other carbohydrate, vitamins (such as biotin, folate, niacin, riboflavin, pantothenic acid, thiamin, vitamin B6, vitamin B12, vitamin D, vitamin E, and vitamin K), and minerals (such as chromium, copper, iodine, magnesium, manganese, molybdenum, phosphorus, potassium, selenium, and zinc).

(Source: "What's On The Nutrition Facts Label," U.S Food and Drug Administration (FDA).)

6. Be A Healthy Role Model

Encourage your friends to practice healthier habits. Share what you do to work through challenges. Keep your computer and TV time to less than 2 hours a day (unless it's school work).

7. Try Something New

Keep healthy eating fun by picking out new foods you've never tried before like lentils, mango, quinoa or kale.

8. Make Moving Part Of Every Event

Being active makes everyone feel good. Aim for 60 minutes of physical activity each day. Move your body often. Dancing, playing active games, walking to school with friends, swimming, and biking are only a few fun ways to be active. Also, try activities that target the muscles in your arms and legs.

9. Include All Food Groups Daily

Use MyPlate as your guide to include all food groups each day.

10. Everyone Has Different Needs

Get nutrition information based on your age, gender, height, weight, and physical activity level. Use SuperTracker (www.supertracker.usda.gov) to find your calorie level, choose the foods you need, and track progress toward your goals.

Choose The Foods You Need To Grow: Ten Tips For Teen Guys

Feed your growing body by making better food choices today as a teen and as you continue to grow into your twenties. Make time to be physically active every day to help you be fit and healthy as you grow.

1. Get Over The Idea Of Magic Foods

There are no magic foods to eat for good health. Teen guys need to eat foods such as vegetables, fruits, whole grains, protein foods, and fat-free or low-fat dairy foods. Choose protein foods like unsalted nuts, beans, lean meats, and fish.

2. Always Hungry?

Whole grains that provide fiber can give you a feeling of fullness and provide key nutrients. Choose half your grains as whole grains. Eat whole-wheat breads, pasta, and brown rice instead of white bread, rice or other refined grains. Also, choose vegetables and fruits when you need to "fill-up."

3. Keep Water Handy

Water is a better option than many other drink choices. Keep a water bottle in your backpack and at your desk to satisfy your thirst. Skip soda, fruit drinks, and energy and sports drinks. They are sugar-sweetened and have few nutrients.

4. Make A List Of Favorite Foods

Like green apples more than red apples? Ask your family food shopper to buy quick-to-eat foods for the fridge like mini-carrots, apples oranges, low-fat cheese slices or yogurt. And also try dried fruit; unsalted nuts; whole-grain breads, cereal, and crackers; and popcorn.

5. Start Cooking Often

Get over being hungry by fixing your own snacks and meals. Learn to make vegetable omelets, bean quesadillas or a batch of spaghetti. Prepare your own food so you can make healthier meals and snacks. Microwaving frozen pizzas doesn't count as home cooking.

6. Skip Foods That Can Add Unwanted Pounds

Cut back on calories by limiting fatty meats like ribs, bacon, and hot dogs. Some foods are just occasional treats like pizza, cakes, cookies, candies, and ice cream. Check out the calorie content of sugary drinks by reading the Nutrition Facts label. Many 12-ounce sodas contain 10 teaspoons of sugar.

7. Learn How Much Food You Need

Teen guys may need more food than most adults, teen girls, and little kids. Go to www.SuperTracker.usda.gov. It shows how much food you need based on your age, height, weight, and activity level. It also tracks progress towards fitness goals.

8. Check Nutrition Facts Labels

To grow, your body needs vitamins and minerals. Calcium and vitamin D are especially important for your growing bones. Read Nutrition Facts labels for calcium. Dairy foods provide the minerals your bones need to grow.

Calcium is needed for our heart, muscles, and nerves to function properly and for blood to clot. Inadequate calcium significantly contributes to the development of osteoporosis. Many published studies show that low calcium intake throughout life is associated with low bone mass and high fracture rates. National nutrition surveys have shown that most people are not getting the calcium they need to grow and maintain healthy bones.

(Source: "Calcium And Vitamin D: Important At Every Age," National Institute of Arthritis and Musculoskeletal and Skin Diseases (NIAMS).)

9. Strengthen Your Muscles

Work on strengthening and aerobic activities. Work out at least 10 minutes at a time to see a better you. However, you need to get at least 60 minutes of physical activity every day.

10. Fill Your Plate Like Myplate

Go to www.ChooseMyPlate.gov for more easy tips and science-based nutrition from the *Dietary Guidelines for Americans* (www.DietaryGuidelines.gov).

Chapter 7

Weighty Issues

What Is A Healthy Weight?[1]

As you enter your teen years, so much is changing in your body (and your mind), that it may be hard for you to know what a healthy weight is.

Sometimes, teenagers think they need to be thinner, even if they are not overweight. You may see models in magazines or on TV who are really skinny, and you may think that you need to lose weight so you can look like them. But many of these models are underweight to a point that is unhealthy.

So how do you find out if you are a healthy weight? One tool that can help tell if you are at a healthy weight for your age and height is the BMI. Talk with your doctor about BMI and your weight. Together, you can decide whether you need to lose weight, gain weight, or stop worrying about your weight.

Body Mass Index (BMI) For Children And Teens[2]

BMI is a measure used to determine childhood overweight and obesity. Overweight is defined as a BMI at or above the 85th percentile and below the 95th percentile for children and teens of the same age and sex. Obesity is defined as a BMI at or above the 95th percentile for children and teens of the same age and sex.

About This Chapter: This chapter includes text excerpted from documents published by three public domain sources. Text under headings marked 1 are excerpted from "A Healthy Weight For Girls" girlshealth.gov, Office on Women's Health (OWH), November 5, 2013. Reviewed September 2017; Text under heading marked 2 is excerpted from "Defining Childhood Obesity," Centers for Disease Control and Prevention (CDC), October 20, 2016; Text under headings marked 3 are excerpted from "Finding A Balance," Centers for Disease Control and Prevention (CDC), November 16, 2016.

BMI is calculated by dividing a person's weight in kilograms by the square of height in meters. For children and teens, BMI is age- and sex-specific and is often referred to as BMI-for-age. A child's weight status is determined using an age- and sex-specific percentile for BMI rather than the BMI categories used for adults. This is because children's body composition varies as they age and varies between boys and girls. Therefore, BMI levels among children and teens need to be expressed relative to other children of the same age and sex.

For example, a 10-year-old boy of average height (56 inches) who weighs 102 pounds would have a BMI of 22.9 kg/m^2. This would place the boy in the 95th percentile for BMI, and he would be considered as obese. This means that the child's BMI is greater than the BMI of 95 percent of 10-year-old boys in the reference population.

Table 7.1. Weight Status Category And Percentile Range

Weight Status Category	Percentile Range
Underweight	Less than the 5th percentile
Normal or Healthy Weight	5th percentile to less than the 85th percentile
Overweight	85th to less than the 95th percentile
Obese	95th percentile or greater

BMI does not measure body fat directly, but research has shown that BMI is correlated with more direct measures of body fat, such as skinfold thickness measurements, bioelectrical impedance, densitometry (underwater weighing), dual energy X-ray absorptiometry (DXA) and other methods. BMI can be considered an alternative to direct measures of body fat. A trained healthcare provider should perform appropriate health assessments in order to evaluate an individual's health status and risks.

Overweight And Obesity[1]

A person who is "overweight" weighs more than is considered healthy. A person who is "obese" has even more extra weight.

Being overweight or obese comes with the possibility of some serious health problems, including a risk of:

- Diabetes

- Heart disease

- Cancer

- Asthma

- Problems with menstruation (periods)

- Strain on your joints

- Sleep problems

What Are Calories?[1]

Calories are a form of energy. The calories in food mean the energy that the food supplies to a person's body. The calories and physical activity mean the energy that your body uses ("burns") to do the activity.

To stay at a healthy weight, you want to take in around the same amount of calories as you use for activity. Are you active a moderate, or medium, amount? (That means something between sitting around a lot and walking more than 3 miles per day.) If so, you probably can eat around 2,000 calories each day.

Caloric Balance Equation[3]

Whether you need to lose weight, maintain your ideal weight, or gain weight, the main message is—calories count! Weight management is all about balancing the number of calories you take in with the number your body uses or "burns off."

- A *calorie* is a unit of energy supplied by food and beverages. A calorie is a calorie regardless of its source. Carbohydrates, fats, sugars, and proteins all contain calories.

- If your body does not use calories, they are stored as fat.

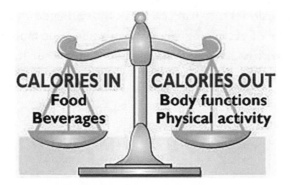

Figure 7.1. Scale Caloric Balance

- *Caloric balance* is like a scale. To remain in balance and maintain your body weight, the calories consumed must be balanced by the calories used in normal body functions, daily activities, and exercise.

Table 7.2. Caloric Balance Equation

If You Are...	Your Caloric Balance Status Is...
Maintaining your weight	"in balance." You are eating roughly the same number of calories that your body is using. Your weight will remain stable.
Gaining weight	"in caloric excess." You are eating more calories than your body is using. You will store these extra calories as fat and you'll gain weight.
Losing weight	"in caloric deficit." You are eating fewer calories than you are using. Your body is pulling from its fat storage cells for energy, so your weight is decreasing.

Balancing Diet And Activity To Lose And Maintain Weight Count, Cut, And Burn Calories[3]

If your body weight has not changed for several months, you are in caloric balance. If you need to gain or lose weight, you'll need to balance your diet and activity level to achieve your goal.

It takes about 3,500 calories to lose a pound of body fat, You can do this by reducing the calories you take in and increasing the calories you burn. An adult can lose 1 to 2 pounds per week by avoiding or burning 500–1000 calories per day.

To learn how many calories you are taking in, write down the foods you eat and the beverages you drink, plus the calories they have, each day. By writing down what you eat and drink, you become more aware of everything you are putting in your mouth. Also, begin writing down your physical activity each day and the length of time you do it.

Chapter 8

Mental Wellness

Your mental health is very important. You will not have a healthy body if you don't also take care of your mind. People depend on you. It's important for you to take care of yourself so that you can do the important things in life—whether it's working, learning, taking care of your family, volunteering, enjoying the outdoors, or whatever is important to you.

Good mental health helps you enjoy life and cope with problems. It offers a feeling of well-being and inner strength. Just as you take care of your body by eating right and exercising, you can do things to protect your mental health. In fact, eating right and exercising can help maintain good mental health. You don't automatically have good mental health just because you don't have mental health illness. You have to work to keep your mind healthy.

> Mental health includes our emotional, psychological, and social well-being. It affects how we think, feel, and act. It also helps determine how we handle stress, relate to others, and make choices. Mental health is important at every stage of life, from childhood and adolescence through adulthood.
>
> *(Source: "What Is Mental Health?" MentalHealth.gov, U.S. Department of Health and Human Services (HHS).)*

About This Chapter: Text in this chapter begins with excerpts from "Mental Health—Good Mental Health," Office on Women's Health (OWH), U.S. Department of Health and Human Services (HHS); March 29, 2010. Reviewed September 2017; Text under the heading "Mental And Emotional Well-Being" is excerpted from "Mental And Emotional Well-Being," Surgeongeneral.gov, U.S. Department of Health and Human Services (HHS), June 18, 2011. Reviewed September 2017; Text under the heading "Being Active Is Good For Your Mental Health" is excerpted from "Fitness—Why Physical Activity Is Important," girlshealth.gov, Office on Women's Health (OWH), June 22, 2015.

Nutrition And Mental Health

The food you eat can have a direct effect on your energy level, physical health, and mood. A "healthy diet" is one that has enough of each essential nutrient, contains many foods from all of the basic food groups, provides the right amount of calories to maintain a healthy weight, and does not have too much fat, sugar, salt, or alcohol.

By choosing foods that can give you steady energy, you can help your body stay healthy. This may also help your mind feel good. The same diet doesn't work for every person. In order to find the best foods that are right for you, talk to your healthcare professional.

Some vitamins and minerals may help with the symptoms of depression. Experts are looking into how a lack of some nutrients—including folate, vitamin B12, calcium, iron, selenium, zinc, and omega-3—may contribute to depression in new mothers. Ask your doctor or another healthcare professional for more information.

Exercise And Mental Health

Regular physical activity is important to the physical and mental health of almost everyone, including older adults. Being physically active can help you continue to do the things you enjoy and stay independent as you age. Regular physical activity over long periods of time can produce long-term health benefits. That's why health experts say that everyone should be active every day to maintain their health.

If you are diagnosed with depression or anxiety, your doctor may tell you to exercise in addition to taking any medications or receiving counseling. This is because exercise has been shown to help with the symptoms of depression and anxiety. Your body makes certain chemicals, called endorphins, before and after you work out. They relieve stress and improve your mood. Exercise can also slow or stop weight gain, which is a common side effect of some medications used to treat mental health disorders.

Sleep And Mental Health

Your mind and body will feel better if you sleep well. Your body needs time every day to rest and heal. If you often have trouble sleeping—either falling asleep, or waking during the night and being unable to get back to sleep—one or several of the following ideas might be helpful to you:

- Go to bed at the same time every night and get up at the same time every morning. Avoid "sleeping in" (sleeping much later than your usual time for getting up). It will make you feel worse.

- Establish a bedtime "ritual" by doing the same things every night for an hour or two before bedtime so your body knows when it is time to go to sleep.

- Avoid caffeine, nicotine, and alcohol.

- Eat on a regular schedule and avoid a heavy meal prior to going to bed. Don't skip any meals.

- Eat plenty of dairy foods and dark green leafy vegetables.

- Exercise daily, but avoid strenuous or invigorating activity before going to bed.

- Play soothing music on a tape or CD that shuts off automatically after you are in bed.

- Try a turkey sandwich and a glass of milk before bedtime to make you feel drowsy.

- Try having a small snack before you go to bed, something like a piece of fruit and a piece of cheese, so you don't wake up hungry in the middle of the night. Have a similar small snack if you awaken in the middle of the night.

- Take a warm bath or shower before going to bed.

- Place a drop of lavender oil on your pillow.

- Drink a cup of herbal chamomile tea before going to bed.

You need to see your doctor if:

- You often have difficulty sleeping and the solutions listed above are not working for you

- You awaken during the night gasping for breath

- Your partner says that your breathing stops when you are sleeping

- You snore loudly

- You wake up feeling like you haven't been asleep

- You fall asleep often during the day

Stress And Mental Health

Stress can happen for many reasons. Stress can be brought about by a traumatic accident, death, or emergency situation. Stress can also be a side effect of a serious illness or disease. There is also stress associated with daily life, the workplace, and family responsibilities. It's hard to stay calm and relaxed in our hectic lives. As women, we have many roles: spouse, mother, caregiver, friend, and/or worker. With all we have going on in our lives, it seems almost impossible to find ways to de-stress. But it's important to find those ways. Your health depends on it.

Common symptoms include:

- Headache

- Sleep disorders

- Difficulty concentrating

- Short-temper

- Upset stomach

- Job dissatisfaction

- Low morale

- Depression

- Anxiety

Remember to always make time for you. It's important to care for yourself. Think of this as an order from your doctor, so you don't feel guilty! No matter how busy you are, you can try to set aside at least 15 minutes each day in your schedule to do something for yourself, like taking a bubble bath, going for a walk, or calling a friend.

Mental And Emotional Well-Being

Mental and emotional well-being is essential to overall health. Positive mental health allows people to realize their full potential, cope with the stresses of life, work productively, and make meaningful contributions to their communities. Early childhood experiences have

Recommendations

1. Promote positive early childhood development, including positive parenting and violence-free homes.

2. Facilitate social connectedness and community engagement across the lifespan.

3. Provide individuals and families with the support necessary to maintain positive mental well-being.

4. Promote early identification of mental health needs and access to quality services.

lasting, measurable consequences later in life; therefore, fostering emotional well-being from the earliest stages of life helps build a foundation for overall health and well-being. Anxiety, mood (e.g., depression), and impulse control disorders are associated with a higher probability of risk behaviors (e.g., tobacco, alcohol and other drug use, risky sexual behavior), intimate partner and family violence, many other chronic and acute conditions (e.g., obesity, diabetes, cardiovascular disease, human immunodeficiency virus (HIV)/sexually transmitted infections (STI)), and premature death.

Being Active Is Good For Your Mental Health

Did you know being physically active can affect how good you feel? It also can affect how well you do your tasks, and even how pleasant you are to be around. That's partly because physical activity gets your brain to make "feel-good" chemicals called endorphins. Regular physical activity may help you by:

- Reducing stress

- Improving sleep

- Boosting your energy

- Reducing symptoms of anxiety and depression

- Increasing your self-esteem

- Making you feel proud for taking good care of yourself

- Improving how well you do at school

Chapter 9

Sleep Is Important For Fitness

Why Is Sleep Important?

Sleep plays a vital role in good health and well-being throughout your life. Getting enough quality sleep at the right times can help protect your mental health, physical health, quality of life, and safety. The way you feel while you're awake depends in part on what happens while you're sleeping. During sleep, your body is working to support healthy brain function and maintain your physical health. In children and teens, sleep also helps support growth and development. The damage from sleep deficiency can occur in an instant (such as a car crash), or it can harm you over time. For example, ongoing sleep deficiency can raise your risk for some chronic health problems. It also can affect how well you think, react, work, learn, and get along with others.

Healthy Brain Function And Emotional Well-Being

Sleep helps your brain work properly. While you're sleeping, your brain is preparing for the next day. It's forming new pathways to help you learn and remember information.

Studies show that a good night's sleep improves learning. Whether you're learning math, how to play the piano, how to perfect your golf swing, or how to drive a car, sleep helps enhance your learning and problem-solving skills. Sleep also helps you pay attention, make decisions, and be creative.

About This Chapter: Text under the heading "Why Is Sleep Important?" is excerpted from "Why Is Sleep Important?" National Heart, Lung, and Blood Institute (NHLBI), June 7, 2017; Text under the heading "Teen Sleep Habits" is excerpted from "Teen Sleep Habits," Centers for Disease Control and Prevention (CDC), October 13, 2011. Reviewed September 2017; Text under the heading "Tips For Better Sleep" is excerpted from "Tips For Better Sleep," Centers for Disease Control and Prevention (CDC), July 15, 2016.

Studies also show that sleep deficiency alters activity in some parts of the brain. If you're sleep deficient, you may have trouble making decisions, solving problems, controlling your emotions and behavior, and coping with change. Sleep deficiency also has been linked to depression, suicide, and risk-taking behavior.

Children and teens who are sleep deficient may have problems getting along with others. They may feel angry and impulsive, have mood swings, feel sad or depressed, or lack motivation. They also may have problems paying attention, and they may get lower grades and feel stressed.

Physical Health

Sleep plays an important role in your physical health. For example, sleep is involved in healing and repair of your heart and blood vessels. Ongoing sleep deficiency is linked to an increased risk of heart disease, kidney disease, high blood pressure, diabetes, and stroke.

Sleep deficiency also increases the risk of obesity. For example, one study of teenagers showed that with each hour of sleep lost, the odds of becoming obese went up. Sleep deficiency increases the risk of obesity in other age groups as well.

Sleep helps maintain a healthy balance of the hormones that make you feel hungry (ghrelin) or full (leptin). When you don't get enough sleep, your level of ghrelin goes up and your level of leptin goes down. This makes you feel hungrier than when you're well-rested.

Sleep also affects how your body reacts to insulin, the hormone that controls your blood glucose (sugar) level. Sleep deficiency results in a higher than normal blood sugar level, which may increase your risk for diabetes.

Sleep also supports healthy growth and development. Deep sleep triggers the body to release the hormone that promotes normal growth in children and teens. This hormone also boosts muscle mass and helps repair cells and tissues in children, teens, and adults. Sleep also plays a role in puberty and fertility.

Your immune system relies on sleep to stay healthy. This system defends your body against foreign or harmful substances. Ongoing sleep deficiency can change the way in which your immune system responds. For example, if you're sleep deficient, you may have trouble fighting common infections.

Daytime Performance And Safety

Getting enough quality sleep at the right times helps you function well throughout the day. People who are sleep deficient are less productive at work and school. They take longer to finish tasks, have a slower reaction time, and make more mistakes. After several nights of losing sleep—even a loss of just 1–2 hours per night—your ability to function suffers as if you haven't slept at all for a day or two. Lack of sleep also may lead to microsleep. Microsleep refers to brief moments of sleep that occur when you're normally awake.

You can't control microsleep, and you might not be aware of it. For example, have you ever driven somewhere and then not remembered part of the trip? If so, you may have experienced microsleep. Even if you're not driving, microsleep can affect how you function. If you're listening to a lecture, for example, you might miss some of the information or feel like you don't understand the point. In reality, though, you may have slept through part of the lecture and not been aware of it.

Some people aren't aware of the risks of sleep deficiency. In fact, they may not even realize that they're sleep deficient. Even with limited or poor-quality sleep, they may still think that they can function well. For example, drowsy drivers may feel capable of driving. Yet, studies show that sleep deficiency harms your driving ability as much as, or more than, being drunk. It's estimated that driver sleepiness is a factor in about 100,000 car accidents each year, resulting in about 1,500 deaths. Drivers aren't the only ones affected by sleep deficiency. It can affect people in all lines of work, including healthcare workers, pilots, students, lawyers, mechanics, and assembly line workers. As a result, sleep deficiency is not only harmful on a personal level, but it also can cause large-scale damage. For example, sleep deficiency has played a role in human errors linked to tragic accidents, such as nuclear reactor meltdowns, grounding of large ships, and aviation accidents.

Teen Sleep Habits
What Should You Do?

Almost 70 percent of high school students are not getting the recommended hours of sleep on school nights, according to a study by the Centers for Disease Control and Prevention (CDC).

Researchers found insufficient sleep (< 8 hours on an average school night) to be associated with a number of unhealthy activities, such as:

- Drinking soda or pop 1 or more times per day (not including diet soda or diet pop)
- Not participating in 60 minutes of physical activity on 5 or more of the past 7 days
- Using computers 3 or more hours each day
- Being in a physical fight 1 or more times

- Cigarette use

- Alcohol use

- Marijuana use

- Current sexual activity

- Feeling sad or hopeless

- Seriously considering attempting suicide

Adolescents not getting sufficient sleep each night may be due to changes in the sleep/wake-cycle as well as everyday activities, such as employment, recreational activities, academic pressures, early school start times, and access to technology.

The National Sleep Foundation (NSF) recommends that teenagers receive between 8.5 hours and 9.25 hours each night.

The following sleep health tips are recommended by the NSF:

- Go to bed at the same time each night and rise at the same time each morning.

- Make sure your bedroom is a quiet, dark, and relaxing environment, which is neither too hot or too cold.

- Make sure your bed is comfortable and use it only for sleeping and not for other activities, such as reading, watching TV, or listening to music. Remove all TVs, computers, and other "gadgets" from the bedroom.

- Avoid large meals a few hours before bedtime.

If your sleep problems persist or if they interfere with how you feel or function during the day, you should seek the assistance of a physician or other health professional. Before visiting your physician, consider keeping a diary of your sleep habits for about ten days to discuss at the visit.

Include the following in your sleep diary, when you:

- Go to bed.

- Go to sleep.

- Wake up.

- Get out of bed.

- Take naps.

- Exercise.

- Consume alcohol and how much.

- Consume caffeinated beverages and how much.

Tips For Better Sleep

Good sleep habits (sometimes referred to as "sleep hygiene") can help you get a good night's sleep. Some habits that can improve your sleep health:

- Be consistent. Go to bed at the same time each night and get up at the same time each morning, including on the weekends.

- Make sure your bedroom is quiet, dark, relaxing, and at a comfortable temperature.

- Remove electronic devices, such as TVs, computers, and smartphones, from the bedroom.

- Avoid large meals, caffeine, and alcohol before bedtime.

- Get some exercise. Being physically active during the day can help you fall asleep more easily at night.

Part Two
Making And Maintaining A Fitness Plan

Chapter 10

Tips For Getting Started On A Path To Fitness

Are you new to physical activity? Start with small steps, like getting off the bus a couple of blocks early or taking the stairs instead of the elevator.

Do you think, "I don't have time to workout" or "Exercise is too boring!"? You may have lots of reasons not to be active.

How To Make A Fitness Plan

Use the three steps and tips below to make a personal fitness plan that's right for you.

1. Set Goals

- **Be specific.** Saying something like "I'll be active three days a week" works better than "I'll exercise more."

- **Be realistic.** If you try to increase your activity a lot all at once, you may get overwhelmed.

- **Go slow.** Try tackling just one goal at a time instead of several. After sticking with your goal for a couple of weeks, see if you can add another one.

2. Pick Small Steps

- **Break your goal into smaller steps.** That way it will feel more doable. If you said "I'll be active three days a week," for example, start by figuring out which days might work.

- **Pick items you enjoy.** You are more likely to stick with activities you enjoy. If you decide to walk, for example, ask a friend to join you to make it more fun.

About This Chapter: This chapter includes text excerpted from "Getting Started And Staying Active," girlshealth. gov, Office on Women's Health (OWH), March 27, 2015.

- **Enter a few steps on your calendar.** Pick days. That way you won't forget and you'll make sure you have enough time.

3. Monitor Your Progress

- **Check your list.** See what you've done in the past week.

- **Did you skip a lot of your fitness time?** Don't give up! Creating new habits does not happen fast. This is a chance to see what gets in your way and then find solutions. For example, maybe you need to exercise in the morning instead of at night.

- **Did you succeed a lot of the time?** Celebrate! Reward yourself! Tell your friends and family! You might inspire them.

Making Physical Activity Fun

Here are some ways to beat boredom:

- **Join a team.** Playing a sport can be a great way to make friends.

- **Walk or ride a bike to school.** It's good for you and for the environment.

- **Be active while doing something you like.** Maybe march in place while you watch TV or listen to some energizing music.

- **Join a cause.** A walk-a-thon or other fundraiser is a great way to get fit and do something good.

- **Take a class or join a group.** Your local community center may have classes or exercise groups.

- **Try something new.** Try a DVD or take a class to learn some moves. How about yoga, Pilates External link, or martial arts?

Got games? Exercise video games (like you play on Xbox or Wii) that get you moving can add to your fitness routine. But for a good workout, make sure to pick options that use your whole body, such as boxing, dancing, or tennis. Also, try not to let this be your only exercise. (And don't forget to get some fresh air!)

Some people love to be active outside. Some people like walking in the calm of nature, or shooting hoops in the playground.

Some people want to stay inside. Maybe your neighborhood isn't safe, or you hate the cold (or heat). If that's you, here are some options:

- Walk up and down stairs

- March in place

- Jump rope

- Tune in to TV or online exercise programs

- Borrow an exercise DVD from your library

- Clean the house with some extra energy

- Pump up some music and dance

Ways To Get Over Exercise Excuses

If you've not been physically active in a while, you may be wondering how to get started again. Lace up those sneakers and find some motivating ideas here.

Here are some tips to help get you started:

- Look for opportunities to reduce sedentary time and to increase active time. For example, instead of watching TV, try taking a walk after dinner.

- Set aside specific times for physical activity in your schedule to make it part of your daily or weekly routine.

- Start with activities, locations, and times you enjoy. For example, some people might like walking in their neighborhood in the mornings; others might prefer an exercise class at a health club after work.

- Try activities with friends or family members to help with motivation and mutual encouragement.

- Start slowly and work your way up to more physically challenging activities. For many people, walking is a particularly good place to begin.

- When necessary, break up your daily activity goal into smaller amounts of time. For example, you could break the 30-minute a day recommendation into three 10-minute sessions or two 15-minute sessions. Just make sure the shorter sessions are at least 10 minutes long.

(Source: "Getting Started With Physical Activity For A Healthy Weight," Centers for Disease Control and Prevention (CDC).)

Getting Rid Of Excuses

"I am too busy."

- Try different times of the day to see what works best for you.

- Just do a little at a time, aiming for at least 60 minutes by the end of the day.

- See if you can cut out something to make the time for physical activity.

- Try scheduling exercise the same way you plan for other activities and commitments.

- Exercise may be tiring at first, but over time it will give you more energy to do what you need to do.

"Exercise is boring."

- Try different activities. Maybe rollerblading, Pilates, hiking, or dancing are more your speed.

- Add music or friends to liven things up!

- Aim for variety. Do different activities on different days.

"It's hard to stick with it."

- Make a list of the reasons you want to get fit. Look at it often.

- Work out with a friend or family member. You'll be less likely to cancel if someone else is involved.

"I don't have equipment or a health club membership."

- Do activities that don't require a gym, like jumping rope. Be creative. Walk your dog (or borrow a friend's).

- Find out what your community offers. Contact a community center, church, or parks and recreation office. They may have free or lower-cost programs. Maybe a local school has a track or pool. Think about joining a walk-a-thon for a good cause.

- For muscle-building, use canned food. Or use your body weight with activities like sit-ups and push-ups.

"I don't know how."

- Start with activities you already know, like walking or climbing stairs.

- See if you can find a friend who can teach you a skill you want to learn.

- Take a class at a community center or health club.

- Get help by joining a team sport at school.

"I'm going to look bad when I work out."

- We think anyone who is working out looks good! Exercising means you look like someone who cares about her health—and likes to have fun!

- Consider getting started in private first. Close your door and dance, walk up and down stairs, or clean your room with extra energy.

- See if you can get out there anyway. Try to focus on how great you are going to feel, instead of what other people think. Be true to you!

Chapter 11

Fitness Guidelines For Children And Adolescents

Regular physical activity in children and adolescents promotes health and fitness. Compared to those who are inactive, physically active youth have higher levels of cardiorespiratory fitness and stronger muscles. They also typically have lower body fatness. Their bones are stronger, and they may have reduced symptoms of anxiety and depression.

Youth who are regularly active also have a better chance of a healthy adulthood. Children and adolescents don't usually develop chronic diseases, such as heart disease, hypertension, type 2 diabetes, or osteoporosis. However, risk factors for these diseases can begin to develop early in life. Regular physical activity makes it less likely that these risk factors will develop and more likely that children will remain healthy as adults.

Youth can achieve substantial health benefits by doing moderate- and vigorous-intensity physical activity for periods of time that add up to 60 minutes (1 hour) or more each day. This activity should include aerobic activity as well as age-appropriate muscle- and bone–strengthening activities. Although current science is not complete, it appears that, as with adults, the total amount of physical activity is more important for achieving health benefits than is any one component (frequency, intensity, or duration) or specific mix of activities (aerobic, muscle-strengthening, bone strengthening).

Even so, bone-strengthening activities remain especially important for children and young adolescents because the greatest gains in bone mass occur during the years just before and during puberty. In addition, the majority of peak bone mass is obtained by the end of adolescence.

About This Chapter: This chapter includes text excerpted from "Chapter 3: Active Children And Adolescents," Office of Disease Prevention and Health Promotion (ODPHP), U.S. Department of Health and Human Services (HHS), September 1, 2017.

This chapter provides physical activity guidance for children and adolescents aged 6 to 17, and focuses on physical activity beyond baseline activity.

Key Guidelines For Children And Adolescents

- Children and adolescents should do 60 minutes (1 hour) or more of physical activity daily.

  - **Aerobic:** Most of the 60 or more minutes a day should be either moderate- or vigorous-intensity aerobic physical activity, and should include vigorous-intensity physical activity at least 3 days a week.

  - **Muscle-strengthening:** As part of their 60 or more minutes of daily physical activity, children and adolescents should include muscle-strengthening physical activity on at least 3 days of the week.

  - **Bone-strengthening:** As part of their 60 or more minutes of daily physical activity, children and adolescents should include bone-strengthening physical activity on at least 3 days of the week.

It is important to encourage young people to participate in physical activities that are appropriate for their age, that are enjoyable, and that offer variety.

Types Of Activity

The *Physical Activity Guidelines for Americans* (PAG or the Guidelines) for children and adolescents focus on three types of activity: aerobic, muscle-strengthening, and bone-strengthening. Each type has important health benefits.

- **Aerobic activities** are those in which young people rhythmically move their large muscles. Running, hopping, skipping, jumping rope, swimming, dancing, and bicycling are all examples of aerobic activities. Aerobic activities increase cardiorespiratory fitness. Children often do activities in short bursts, which may not technically be aerobic activities.

- **Muscle-strengthening activities** make muscles do more work than usual during activities of daily life. This is called "overload," and it strengthens the muscles. Muscle-strengthening activities can be unstructured and part of play, such as playing on playground equipment, climbing trees, and playing tug-of-war. Or these activities can be structured, such as lifting weights or working with resistance bands.

- **Bone-strengthening activities** produce a force on the bones that promotes bone growth and strength. This force is commonly produced by impact with the ground. Running, jumping rope, basketball, tennis, and hopscotch are all examples of bone strengthening activities. As these examples illustrate, bone-strengthening activities can also be aerobic and muscle-strengthening.

Other things that you can do:

- Choosing activities that work all the different parts of the body, including your core (muscles around your trunk and pelvis). Good core strength improves balance and stability and helps to prevent lower back injury.

- Choosing activities that you enjoy. It's easier to make exercise a regular part of your life if you have fun doing it.

- Exercising safely, with proper equipment, to prevent injuries. Also, listen to your body and don't overdo it.

- Giving yourself goals. The goals should challenge you, but also be realistic. It's also helpful to reward yourself when you reach your goals. The rewards could be something big, like new workout gear, or something smaller, such as movie tickets.

(Source: "Exercise And Physical Fitness," MedlinePlus, National Institutes of Health (NIH).)

How Age Influences Physical Activity In Children And Adolescents

Children and adolescents should meet the Guidelines by doing activity that is appropriate for their age. Their natural patterns of movement differ from those of adults. For example, children are naturally active in an intermittent way, particularly when they do unstructured active play. During recess and in their free play and games, children use basic aerobic and bone-strengthening activities, such as running, hopping, skipping, and jumping, to develop movement patterns and skills. They alternate brief periods of moderate- and vigorous-intensity physical activity with brief periods of rest. Any episode of moderate- or vigorous–intensity physical activity, however brief, counts toward the Guidelines.

Children also commonly increase muscle strength through unstructured activities that involve lifting or moving their body weight or working against resistance. Children don't usually do or need formal muscle-strengthening programs, such as lifting weights.

As children grow into adolescents, their patterns of physical activity change. They are able to play organized games and sports and are able to sustain longer periods of activity. But they still commonly do intermittent activity, and no period of moderate- or vigorous-intensity activity is too short to count toward the Guidelines.

Adolescents may meet the Guidelines by doing free play, structured programs, or both. Structured exercise programs can include aerobic activities, such as playing a sport, and muscle-strengthening activities, such as lifting weights, working with resistance bands, or using body weight for resistance (such as push-ups, pull-ups, and sit-ups). Muscle-strengthening activities count if they involve a moderate to high level of effort and work the major muscle groups of the body: legs, hips, back, abdomen, chest, shoulders, and arms.

Levels Of Intensity For Aerobic Activity

Children and adolescents can meet the Guidelines by doing a combination of moderate- and vigorous intensity aerobic physical activities or by doing only vigorous-intensity aerobic physical activities. Youth should not do only moderate-intensity activity. It's important to include vigorous-intensity activities because they cause more improvement in cardiorespiratory fitness.

The intensity of aerobic physical activity can be defined on either an absolute or a relative scale. Either scale can be used to monitor the intensity of aerobic physical activity:

- **Absolute intensity** is based on the rate of energy expenditure during the activity, without taking into account a person's cardiorespiratory fitness.

- **Relative intensity** uses a person's level of cardiorespiratory fitness to assess level of effort.

Relative intensity describes a person's level of effort relative to his or her fitness. As a rule of thumb, on a scale of 0 to 10, where sitting is 0 and the highest level of effort possible is 10, moderate-intensity activity is a 5 or 6. Young people doing moderate-intensity activity will notice that their hearts are beating faster than normal and they are breathing harder than normal. Vigorous-intensity activity is at a level of 7 or 8. Youth doing vigorous-intensity activity will feel their heart beating much faster than normal and they will breathe much harder than normal.

When adults supervise children, they generally can't ascertain a child's heart or breathing rate. But they can observe whether a child is doing an activity which, based on absolute energy expenditure, is considered to be either moderate or vigorous. For example, a child walking briskly to school is doing moderate-intensity activity. A child running on the playground is doing vigorous-intensity activity.

Moderate-Intensity Aerobic

- Active recreation, such as hiking, skateboarding, rollerblading
- Bicycle riding
- Brisk walking

Vigorous-Intensity Aerobic

- Active games involving running and chasing, such as tag
- Bicycle riding
- Jumping rope
- Martial arts, such as karate
- Running
- Sports such as soccer, ice or field hockey, basketball, swimming, tennis
- Cross-country skiing

Muscle-Strengthening

- Games such as tug-of-war
- Modified push-ups (with knees on the floor)
- Resistance exercises using body weight or resistance bands
- Rope or tree climbing
- Sit-ups (curl-ups or crunches)
- Swinging on playground equipment/bars

Bone-Strengthening

- Games such as hopscotch
- Hopping, skipping, jumping
- Jumping rope
- Running
- Sports such as gymnastics, basketball, volleyball, tennis

Note: Some activities, such as bicycling, can be moderate or vigorous intensity, depending upon level of effort.

Physical Activity And Healthy Weight

Regular physical activity in children and adolescents promotes a healthy body weight and body composition. Exercise training in overweight or obese youth can improve body composition by reducing overall levels of fatness as well as abdominal fatness. Research studies report that fatness can be reduced by regular physical activity of moderate to vigorous intensity 3 to 5 times a week, for 30 to 60 minutes.

Meeting The Guidelines

American youth vary in their physical activity participation. Some don't participate at all, others participate in enough activity to meet the Guidelines, and some exceed the Guidelines.

One practical strategy to promote activity in youth is to replace inactivity with activity whenever possible. For example, where appropriate and safe, young people should walk or bicycle to school instead of riding in a car. Rather than just watching sporting events on television, young people should participate in age-appropriate sports or games.

- **Children and adolescents who do not meet the Guidelines** should slowly increase their activity in small steps and in ways that they enjoy. A gradual increase in the number of days and the time spent being active will help reduce the risk of injury.

- **Children and adolescents who meet the Guidelines** should continue being active on a daily basis and, if appropriate, become even more active. Evidence suggests that even more than 60 minutes of activity every day may provide additional health benefits.

- **Children and adolescents who exceed the Guidelines** should maintain their activity level and vary the kinds of activities they do to reduce the risk of overtraining or injury.

Children and adolescents with disabilities are more likely to be inactive than those without disabilities. Youth with disabilities should work with their healthcare provider to understand the types and amounts of physical activity appropriate for them. When possible, children and adolescents with disabilities should meet the Guidelines. When young people are not able to participate in appropriate physical activities to meet the Guidelines, they should be as active as possible and avoid being inactive.

Chapter 12

A Formula For Fitness

The Overload Principle

The overload principle states that when a system of the body is exercised at a level above that at which it normally operates, the system will adapt and function more efficiently. In strength training, the use of heavy resistances, i.e., resistances exceeding those normally encountered, forces the muscle to contract at maximal or near maximal levels and thus stimulates the physiological adaptations that lead to increases in both muscular strength and size. As a muscle increases in strength, the initial training resistance ceases to overload the exercising muscle and thus becomes ineffective for producing additional strength gains. Continued work with this resistance will enable the participant to maintain a constant level of strength but will not produce additional increases in strength. Further increases in strength require that the muscle be overloaded throughout the course of the strength training program. The process of periodically overloading the muscle as it adapts to the previous workload is called progressive resistance training.

Research indicates that muscular strength can be increased through a variety of training methods. The key to muscular development; however, is the intensity of the work required during the exercise session. In order for training to occur, the overload principle must be satisfied. The principle of progressive resistance exercise implies that strength cannot be increased

About This Chapter: Text beginning with the heading "The Overload Principle" is excerpted from "Astronaut Training Manual," National Aeronautics and Space Administration (NASA), February 8, 2017; Text beginning with the heading "Jump Start Your Routine" is excerpted from "Session 13: Jump Start Your Activity Plan," Centers for Disease Control and Prevention (CDC), April 20, 2012. Reviewed September 2017; Text under the heading "Be F.I.T.T." is excerpted from "FITT—Frequency, Intensity, Time, And Type Of Activity," U.S. Department of Veterans Affairs (VA), August 23, 2012. Reviewed September 2017.

by lifting light to moderate workloads. The muscle must constantly attempt the momentarily impossible. Attempting to lift maximal or near maximal loads causes the body to utilize its reserve ability. The utilization of this reserve ability is the essential factor in stimulating muscular growth.

Increasing The Workload

In most strength training routines, the participant performs a set number of repetitions of a given exercise with a predetermined workload. A typical example for an exercise utilizing the bench press maneuver might consist of 10 repetitions with 100 pounds of weight. This 100-pound workload is referred to as the 10-RM (10 repetition maximum). A 10-RM is a load that can be lifted correctly only ten times before fatigue sets in. During each training session, the participant should lift the 100-pound load at least 10 times. As the body adjusts to the workload, muscular strength increases and the participant is able to perform more than 10 repetitions with the 100-pound load. The participant should now strive to lift the 100-pound load as many times as possible during each workout. Whenever it is possible to lift the 100-pound load 14 times, the load should be increased by 5 to 10 pounds or until only 10 repetitions can be completed. This process should be repeated throughout training to ensure that the muscle is always adequately overloaded.

Jump Start Your Routine

After a while, your activity routine might become a little boring. Boredom is a problem because it may cause you to slip back into old habits. It is important to do something to keep your routine fresh and fun. Find ways to jump start your activity routine, giving it new energy. This will also help you to maintain your weight goal.

Adding Variety

You may choose not to do the same activity day in and day out, every season of the year. You are making lifelong changes, and being active is something you will be doing for the rest of your life. Build some variety into your routine, and find ways to make it fun.

Improving Your Aerobic Fitness

As you increase your aerobic activity, you will also improve your aerobic fitness. As you exercise your heart, it will become stronger over time. As your heart becomes stronger, you will notice that it is easier for you to do things, like walking up stairs, or running.

Be F.I.T.T.

What It Means

F.I.T.T. stands for—Frequency, Intensity, Time, and Type of Activity.

When you put a lot of effort into increasing physical activity, you want results! Whether you are a beginner or have experience, FITT will help you build your physical activity program. By following FITT, you are striving to manage your weight and improve your health.

Frequency

How often are you active?

Everyone:

- Be active 5 or more days of the week.

- Start slowly and gradually increase your physical activity.

Beginners:

- Start with 2–3 days of aerobic activity (activity that increases your heart rate). Gradually increase to at least 5 days/week.

Experienced:

- Continue with aerobic activity 5+ days/week.

- Add in 2 days (Tuesday, Thursday) of strength training.

Intensity

How hard are your heart and muscles working?

Everyone (including Beginners):

- Always warm-up, cool-down, and stretch.

- Be active at a moderate intensity (like a brisk walk or gardening).

- Be active at a rate that allows you to talk.

- Slow down if you have trouble breathing or if you can't catch your breath.

- You should stretch after aerobic or strength training. A stretch should never be painful. Some discomfort is normal. You want to feel a slight pull of the muscle.

Experienced:

- Build intensity for aerobic exercise by increasing speed (fast/sprint walk for 30 seconds followed by 1 minute brisk walk) and/or incline/resistance (hills on treadmill, greater workload on bike).

- Increase intensity for strength training by adding weight or only resting 30 seconds between sets.

Time

How long are you active?

Everyone:

- Try to stay active for at least 10 minutes without stopping. Remember, some activity is better than no activity. It is okay to build up to 10 minutes.

- Aim for a total of at least 30 minutes of activity throughout the day. For weight loss, increase this to 60 minutes per day.

- Set a goal for the week based on total minutes of physical activity.

- Increase the length of time you are active before increasing the intensity of the activity.

- There are no time goals for strength training.

- You should stretch after aerobic or strength activity. For muscles that were used, hold each stretch for 15–30 seconds. Repeating stretches will increase flexibility.

Type

What are you doing?

Everyone:

- All types of physical activity are important...so mix it up.
- Aerobic–walking, bicycling, dancing, swimming, mowing the lawn.
- Strength–carrying wood, lifting dumbbells.
- Flexibility–seated stretches, yoga.

Chapter 13

Choosing The Right Type Of Physical Activity

How Can Physical Activity Improve My Health?

The *Physical Activity Guidelines for Americans* state that an active lifestyle can lower your risk of early death from a variety of causes. There is strong evidence that regular physical activity can also lower your risk of:

- Heart disease

- Stroke

- High blood pressure

- Unhealthy cholesterol levels

- Type 2 diabetes

- Metabolic syndrome

- Colon cancer

- Breast cancer

- Falls

- Depression

Regular activity can help prevent unhealthy weight gain and also help with weight loss, when combined with lower calorie intake. If you are overweight or obese, losing weight can

About This Chapter: This chapter includes text excerpted from "Physical Activity," Office on Women's Health (OWH), U.S. Department of Health and Human Services (HHS), June 12, 2017.

lower your risk for many diseases. Being overweight or obese increases your risk of heart disease, high blood pressure, stroke, type 2 diabetes, breathing problems, osteoarthritis, gallbladder disease, sleep apnea (breathing problems while sleeping), and some cancers.

Regular physical activity can also improve your cardiorespiratory (heart, lungs, and blood vessels) and muscular fitness.

Physical activity may also help:

- Improve functional health
- Reduce waistline size
- Lower risk of hip fracture
- Lower risk of lung cancer
- Lower risk of endometrial cancer
- Maintain weight after weight loss
- Increase bone density
- Improve sleep quality

Does The Type Of Physical Activity I Choose Matter?

Yes! Engaging in different types of physical activity is important to overall physical fitness. Your fitness routine should include aerobic and strength-training activities, and may also include stretching activities.

Aerobic Activities

These activities move large muscles in your arms, legs, and hips over and over again. Examples include walking, jogging, bicycling, swimming, and tennis.

Strength-Training Activities

These activities increase the strength and endurance of your muscles. Examples of strength-training activities include working out with weight machines, free weights, and resistance bands. (A resistance band looks like a giant rubber band. You can buy one at a sporting goods store.) Push-ups and sit-ups are examples of strength-training activities you can do without any equipment. You also can use soup cans to work out your arms.

Aim to do strength-training activities at least twice a week. In each strength-training session, you should do 8 to 10 different activities using the different muscle groups throughout your body, such as the muscles in your abdomen, chest, arms, and legs. Repeat each activity 8 to 12 times, using a weight or resistance that will make you feel tired. When you do strength-training activities, slowly increase the amount of weight or resistance that you use. Also, allow one day in between sessions to avoid excess strain on your muscles and joints.

Stretching

Stretching improves flexibility, allowing you to move more easily. This will make it easier for you to reach down to tie your shoes or look over your shoulder when you back the car out of your driveway. You should do stretching activities after your muscles are warmed up—for example, after strength training. Stretching your muscles before they are warmed up may cause injury.

How Much Physical Activity Should I Do?

Health benefits are gained by doing the following each week:

- 2 hours and 30 minutes of moderate-intensity aerobic physical activity or
- 1 hour and 15 minutes of vigorous-intensity aerobic physical activity or
- A combination of moderate and vigorous-intensity aerobic physical activity and
- Muscle-strengthening activities on 2 or more days

This physical activity should be in addition to your routine activities of daily living, such as cleaning or spending a few minutes walking from the parking lot to your office.

Moderate Activity

During moderate-intensity activities you should notice an increase in your heart rate, but you should still be able to talk comfortably. An example of a moderate-intensity activity is walking on a level surface at a brisk pace (about 3 to 4 miles per hour). Other examples include ballroom dancing, leisurely bicycling, moderate housework, and waiting tables.

Vigorous Activity

If your heart rate increases a lot and you are breathing so hard that it is difficult to carry on a conversation, you are probably doing vigorous-intensity activity. Examples of vigorous-intensity activities include jogging, bicycling fast or uphill, singles tennis, and pushing a hand mower.

Physical Activity Behaviors Of Young People

- Only 21.6 percent of 6 to 19-year-old children and adolescents in the Unites States attained 60 or more minutes of moderate-to-vigorous physical activity on at least 5 days per week.

- Only 27.1 percent of high school students participate in at least 60 minutes per day of physical activity on all 7 days of the week.

- In 2015, 53.4 percent of high school students participated in muscle strengthening exercises (e.g., push-ups, sit-ups, weight lifting) on 3 or more days during the week.

- In 2015, 51.6 percent of high school students attended physical education classes in an average week, and only 29.8 percent of high school students attended physical education classes daily.

(Source: "Physical Activity Facts," Centers for Disease Control and Prevention (CDC).)

How Can I Prevent Injuries When I Work Out?

Being physically active is safe if you are careful. Take these steps to prevent injury:

- If you're not active at all or have a health problem, start your program with short sessions (5 to 10 minutes) of physical activity and build up to your goal. (Be sure to ask a doctor before you start if you have a health problem.)

- Use safety equipment such as a helmet for bike riding or supportive shoes for walking or jogging.

- Start every workout with a warm-up. If you plan to walk at a brisk pace, start by walking at an easy pace for 5 to 10 minutes. When you're done working out, do the same thing until your heart rate returns to normal.

- Drink plenty of fluids when you are physically active, even if you are not thirsty.

- Use sunscreen when you are outside.

- Always bend forward from the hips, not the waist. If you keep your back straight, you're probably bending the right way. If your back "humps," that's probably wrong.

- Stop your activity if you feel very out of breath, dizzy, nauseous, or have pain. If you feel tightness or pain in your chest, or you feel faint or have trouble breathing, stop the activity right away and talk to your doctor.

Exercise should not hurt or make you feel really tired. You might feel some soreness, a little discomfort, or a bit weary. But you should not feel pain. In fact, in many ways, being active will probably make you feel better.

Chapter 14

Health Clubs And Fitness Friends

Fitness Centers In The United States

Getting fit and staying fit is a state of mind and an entrepreneurial opportunity. According to IHRSA (International Health, Racquet, and Sportsclub Association), in the beginning of 2015 there were almost 35,500 U.S. Health clubs, which was up 6.4 percent over 2014. In 2014, this accounted for a total U.S. industry revenue of over $24 billion!

The success of the fitness center industry has been fueled by many factors—not the least of which is the growing trend among the 80 million plus baby boomers who see staying fit and healthy as an absolute necessity and daily routine. Also, attrition has gone down because members are reluctant to give up their health club memberships choosing to save money instead on big ticket items such as vacations—reaffirming the fact that "buying" fitness is no longer perceived as a luxury item but a fundamental part of our everyday lives.

Having A Fitness Buddy

Having an exercise buddy can be a fun way to achieve your goals. Many people say they keep active, even on days when it isn't so easy, because they know someone else is counting on them.

About This Chapter: Text under the heading "Fitness Centers In The United States" is excerpted from "6 Steps For Opening A Fitness Center," Small Business Administration (SBA), December 23, 2015; Text under the heading "Having A Fitness Buddy" is excerpted from "Making An Exercise Buddy Agreement," Go4Life, National Institutes of Health (NIH), March 27, 2015; Text under the heading "Five Ways Of Staying Fit With Friends And Family" is excerpted from "5 Friend & Family Fitness Activities To Try Today!" Smokefree.gov, U.S. Department of Health and Human Services (HHS), November 29, 2012. Reviewed September 2017; Text under the heading "Engaging Fitness In The Community" is excerpted from "Engaging Fitness In The Community," U.S. Department of Health and Human Services (HHS), June 7, 2012. Reviewed September 2017.

Make A Plan

Making a plan together is a great way to help you both stay on track. You may even want to put your goals in writing in the form of a friendly "pledge" or agreement. You can use the questions on this form, or adapt it to meet your needs. Print out two copies and fill them out together. Then, to make it "official," both of you should sign them and keep a copy.

Use The Buddy System

Whatever physical activity you choose to engage in can become more enjoyable when a friend or two is doing it alongside you. Having a friend or a group involved helps keep you motivated, and that can give you a boost whenever you're lagging. Knowing that friends are depending on you to meet them for your activity is just the thing to help get you out of the house and keep you going.

(Source: "Physical Fitness—Get Physical," Federal Occupational Health (FOH), U.S. Department of Health and Human Services (HHS).)

Review Your Progress

Refer back to your agreement at a set time to see how things are going. Over time, you'll learn more about what really motivates you and how you can help your friend. Update your agreement regularly so that both of you can continue to go for life!

A Sample Exercise Buddy Agreement

What are two short-term goals you'd both like to achieve during the next month?

Be specific. For example, find out about an exercise class in your area.

What are two long-term goals you'd both like to achieve in the next 6 months?

For example, by this time next year, I'll be able to walk a mile three times a week.

We pledge to support and motivate each other in the following way.

For example, if you stick to your agreement, I'll treat you to coffee or do a household chore for you.

We agree to check our progress and update our goals in:

For example, in 4 weeks on February 11.

Quick Tip

Don't forget to build rewards into your plan. For each goal you reach, treat yourself to something special.

Five Ways Of Staying Fit With Friends And Family

Feeling like there is no way to squeeze in exercise and maintain a social life? Do both—together! Being active with friends and family can be a fun way to get moving. You'll be a great role model, and it's a great way to help the important people in your life live healthy, active lives.

There are lots of ways to be active with friends and family. Try some of these suggestions.

1. **Play!** Swim, toss a ball, or dance to your favorite tunes. Friends and family who play together stay healthy together. If your kids play sports, practice with them! It shows them that you care and is a great way to be active as a family.

2. **Check out your neighborhood!** Walk the dog, go on a bike ride, or head to the park.

3. **Celebrate!** Celebrate special occasions—like birthdays or anniversaries—with something active, like a hike, a volleyball or soccer game, or playing Frisbee.

4. **Ditch your wheels!** If you have to drive, find a spot at the far end of the parking lot. Want to add in some fun? Count the number of steps it takes you to get to the entrance, and try to park farther away next time.

5. **Give back!** Train with friends or family for a charity walk or fun run for a cause or issue that you feel passionate about supporting.

Try This! Give yourself and your friends and family a healthier lifestyle. Choose one day this week to do something active with your loved ones!

Engaging Fitness In The Community

Heading out to engage in physical activity often is easier for people when they can join with others in groups, and support and motivate each other. By engaging communities in physical activity, you can help people share knowledge about the benefits of physical activity, develop awareness about opportunities to be physically active, and overcome barriers and negative attitudes that may exist about exercise.

The U.S. Preventive Service Task Force (USPSTF) recommends several initiatives that communities can adopt to successfully encourage and increase amounts of physical activity, in order to help manage and mitigate chronic health diseases, high blood pressure, and cholesterol. Community access to opportunities for physical activity is extremely important. Building walking trails, pools, fields, and gyms help provide citizens with more opportunities to exercise. Reducing fees for facilities access and providing low or no-cost programming and coaching also helps eliminate barriers to exercise. Simply placing motivational signs by elevators and escalators can remind residents and office workers to use nearby stairs in order to improve health and promote weight management. Community wide media campaigns through television, radio, and newspapers promote screenings and educational workshops at worksites, schools and other community locations. Social support interventions in the community including buddy systems, group walks, and fitness classes also help steer physical behavior in a positive direction while strengthening community bonds and friendships.

There are many cities throughout the country that are making enormous efforts to foster physical activity development and awareness in their communities. Residents are given tools to help attain active lifestyle goals through access to fitness equipment, trails, and online support groups.

Chapter 15

Selecting A Fitness Facility

If you're looking to get in shape, a membership at a gym, fitness center, health spa, or sports club could be a good option. But joining a gym often means signing a contract, and not all contracts are the same. To avoid a problem down the road, find out more about the business and what you're committing to before you sign up. People have told the Federal Trade Commission (FTC) about high-pressure sales tactics, misrepresentations about facilities and services, broken cancellation policies, and lost membership fees when gyms go out of business.

Check Out The Facilities

Plan a visit at a time you would normally be using the gym to see how crowded it is, whether the facilities are clean and well-maintained, and whether the equipment is in good shape. Ask about the:

- **Number of members.** Many gyms set no membership limits. It might not be crowded when you visit, but be packed during peak hours or after a membership drive.

- **Hours of operation.** Do they suit your schedule? Some fitness centers restrict men's use to certain days and women's to others. Some may limit lower-cost memberships to certain hours.

- **Instructors and trainers.** Some places hire trainers and instructors who have special qualifications. If you're looking for professionals to help you, ask about their qualifications and how long they've been on the staff.

About This Chapter: This chapter includes text excerpted from "Joining A Gym," Federal Trade Commission (FTC), July 2012. Reviewed September 2017.

- **Classes.** Will you need to pay extra for certain activities, or are they included in your membership fees?

Know What You're Agreeing To

Some gyms will ask you to join—and pay—the first time you visit and will offer incentives like special rates to get you to sign on the spot. It's best to wait a few days before deciding. Take the contract home and read it carefully. Before you sign, find out:

Is Everything The Salesperson Promised Written In The Contract?

If a problem comes up after you join, the contract is what counts. If something isn't written in the contract, it's going to be difficult to prove your case.

Is There A "Cooling-Off" Or Trial Period?

Some gyms give customers several days to reconsider after they've signed a contract. Others might let you join for a trial period. Even if it costs a little more each month, if you're not enjoying the membership or using it as much as you planned, you will have saved yourself years of payments.

Can You Cancel Your Membership Or Get A Refund?

What happens if you need to cancel your membership because of a move or an injury, or if you find you just aren't using it? Will they refund your money? Knowing the gym's cancellation policies is especially important if you choose a long-term membership.

What happens if the gym goes out of business? You can check with your state Attorney General to see what your rights are according to your state's laws.

Is The Price Right?

Break down the cost to weekly and even daily figures to get a better idea of what you will pay to use the facility. Include possible finance charges if you pay by credit. Can you afford it?

If you signed up for a special introductory rate, make sure you know the terms of your contract once the discounted rate ends.

Find Out What Other People Think

Search For Reviews Online

Do a search online to see what other people are saying about the location you're interested in. You might search the name of the gym with words like "reviews" or "complaints." Are people having the same kinds of issues with their contracts or the facilities?

Check For Complaints And Find Out Your Rights

Contact your state Attorney General or local consumer protection office to find out whether state laws regulate health club memberships, and whether the office has gotten any complaints about the business.

Chapter 16

Exercise Caution Before Spending Money On Fitness Products

When daily trips to the gym aren't possible or gym memberships seem a little too expensive, home exercise equipment might seem like a good alternative. But before you spring for new equipment, make sure you're not buying the fitness fiction of quick, easy results. When shopping, look for equipment that suits your lifestyle and budget, and shop around to get the best price.

What The Ads Say

Home exercise equipment can be a great way to shape up—but only if you use it regularly. Ads promising quick, easy results are selling a line, not a reality. Here are some claims to watch for:

It's quick, easy, and effortless. Whether they're promoting shoes, clothing, or equipment, some advertisers say their products offer a quick, easy way to shape up and lose weight—without sound science to back it up. There's no such thing as a no-work, no-sweat way to a fit, healthy body. To get the benefits of exercise, you have to do the work.

We promise to fix your problem areas. Promises that you can effortlessly burn a spare tire or melt fat from your hips and thighs are tempting, but spot reduction—losing weight in a specific place—takes regular exercise that still works the whole body to burn extra calories.

Look at these before-and-after photos. They may be "satisfied customers," but their experiences may not reflect the results most users get. And celebrity endorsements? They're no proof the product will work as claimed, either. As for the chiseled models in the ads, is that

About This Chapter: This chapter includes text excerpted from "Tips For Buying Exercise Equipment," Federal Trade Commission (FTC), July 2012. Reviewed September 2017.

six-pack the result of the product they're promoting, months in the gym and years of healthy habits, or an altered photo?

What To Do Before You Buy Exercise Equipment

You've done your job and looked at any claims with a skeptical, savvy eye. But you're not quite finished. Before you buy any equipment, here are a few tips to make sure your new gear won't wind up collecting dust:

Start working out. Don't expect the equipment to change your habits. Are you ready to act on your good intentions? If you're not active already, start now.

Find the right equipment. Take a test drive. Before you buy, give different equipment a test drive at a local gym, recreation center, retailer, or even a friend's place.

Read reviews. Check out consumer and fitness magazines that rate exercise equipment to get an idea of how a product performs, and whether it's likely to help you achieve your goal, whether it's building strength, increasing flexibility, improving endurance, or enhancing your health. You also can check out user reviews online. Just don't put all your trust in any one review. Try typing the product or manufacturer's name into a search engine, along with terms like "complaint" or "problem."

Find the right price. Find out the *real* cost. Some companies advertise "three easy payments of $49.95." Break out the calculator and figure out what you'll really pay. Don't forget sales tax and shipping or delivery charges. Find out about warranties, and whether shipping or restocking fees apply if you decide to send it back.

Shop around. That one-of-a-kind fitness product may be available at a better price from a local store, or you might get a better deal online. Factor in delivery costs.

Part Three
Exercise Fundamentals

Chapter 17

Kinds Of Exercise

Exercise and physical activity fall into four basic categories—endurance, strength, balance, and flexibility. Most people tend to focus on one activity or type of exercise and think they're doing enough. Each type is different, though. Doing them all will give you more benefits. Mixing it up also helps to reduce boredom and cut your risk of injury. Though each type is described separately here, some activities fit into more than one category. For example, many endurance activities also build strength. Strength exercises also help improve balance.

Exercising For Endurance

Endurance, or aerobic, activities increase your breathing and heart rate. They keep your heart, lungs, and circulatory system healthy and improve your overall fitness. As a result, they delay or prevent many diseases that are common in older adults, such as diabetes and heart disease. Building your endurance makes it easier to carry out many of your everyday activities.

- Brisk walking or jogging
- Yard work (mowing, raking, digging)
- Dancing
- Swimming
- Biking
- Climbing stairs or hills

About This Chapter: This chapter includes text excerpted from "Exercising For Endurance," MedlinePlus, National Institutes for Health (NIH), 2012. Reviewed September 2017.

- Playing tennis

- Playing basketball

How Much, How Often

Buildup your endurance gradually. If you haven't been active for a long time, it's important to work your way up over time. Start out with 10 minutes at a time and then gradually buildup.

Try to buildup to at least 150 minutes (2 1/2 hours) of moderate endurance activity a week. Being active at least three days a week is best. Remember, these are goals. Some people will be able to do more. It's important to set realistic goals based on your own health and abilities.

Progressing

When you're ready to do more, buildup the amount of time you spend doing endurance activities first, then buildup the difficulty of your activities. For example, gradually increase your time to 30 minutes over several days to weeks by walking longer distances. Then walk more briskly or up steeper hills.

Safety Tips

- Do a little light activity to warm-up and cool down before and after your endurance activities.

- Be sure to drink plenty of liquids when doing any activity that makes you sweat.

- Dress in layers when exercising outdoors so you can add or remove clothes if you get cold or hot.

- To prevent injuries, be sure to use safety equipment.

- Walk during the day or in well-lit areas at night, and be aware of your surroundings.

Exercising For Strength

Strength exercises make your muscles stronger. Even small increases in strength can make a big difference in your ability to stay independent and carry out everyday activities, such as climbing stairs and carrying groceries. These exercises also are called "strength training" or "resistance training."

- Lifting weights

- Using a resistance band

How Much, How Often

Try to do strength exercises for all of your major muscle groups on two or more days per week for 30-minute sessions each, but don't exercise the same muscle group on any two days in a row.

- Depending on your condition, you might need to start out using 1- or 2-pound weights or no weight at all.

- Use a light weight the first week and then gradually add more weight.

- It should feel somewhere between hard and very hard for you to lift or push the weight. If you can't lift or push a weight 8 times in a row, it's too heavy.

- Take 3 seconds to lift a weight into place, hold for 1 second, and return in 3 seconds.

Exercise Instructions

This exercise for your shoulders can help you put things up on a shelf or take them down more easily.

Targeted muscles:

Shoulders

What you need:

Hand-held weights

Stand with your feet shoulder-width apart.

1. Hold weights straight down at your sides, with palms facing backward.

2. Keeping them straight, breathe out as you raise both arms in front of you to shoulder height.

3. Hold the position for 1 second.

4. Breathe in as you slowly lower arms.

5. Repeat 10–15 times.

6. Rest; then repeat 10–15 more times.

Tip: As you progress, use a heavier weight and alternate arms until you can lift the weight comfortably with both arms.

Safety Tips

- Talk with your doctor if you are unsure about doing a particular exercise, especially if you've had hip or back surgery.

- Don't hold your breath during strength exercises. Holding your breath while straining can cause changes in blood pressure. Breathe in slowly through your nose and breathe out slowly through your mouth.

- Breathe out as you lift or push, and breathe in as you relax.

- For some exercises, you may want to start alternating arms and work your way up to using both arms at the same time.

- To prevent injury, don't jerk or thrust weights. Use smooth, steady movements.

- Muscle soreness lasting a few days and slight fatigue are normal after muscle-building exercises, at least at first. After doing these exercises for a few weeks, you will probably not be sore after your workout.

> ## Stretch Yourself
>
> Stretching can be great for your body. It helps keep you flexible so you can reach, bend, and turn more easily. And if you combine stretching with other activities, like strength exercises, it may also prevent injuries. Some ways to increase flexibility are ballet, yoga, martial arts, or pilates. You also can do stretches for specific parts of your body. Make sure to warm-up first. You just need to walk or jog in place for five to 10 minutes.
>
> *(Source: "Fitness Basics—Types Of Physical Activity," girlshealth.gov, Office on Women's Health (OWH).)*

Exercising For Balance

How Much, How Often

You can do balance exercises almost anytime, anywhere, and as often as you like. Also try lower-body strength exercises because they can help improve your balance. Do the lower-body strength exercises two or more days a week but not on any two days in a row.

Progressing

Challenge yourself as you progress. Start by holding onto a sturdy chair for support. When you are able, try holding onto the chair with only one hand. With time, hold on with only one finger, then with no hands at all. If you are really steady on your feet, try doing the exercise with your eyes closed.

Balance exercises help prevent falls, a common problem in older adults. Many lower-body strength exercises also will improve your balance.

- Standing on one foot

- Heel-to-toe walk

- Tai chi

Exercise Instructions

What you need:

Sturdy chair

You can do this exercise while waiting for the bus or standing in line at the grocery. For an added challenge, you can modify the exercise to improve your balance.

- Stand on one foot behind a sturdy chair, holding on for balance.

- Hold position for up to 10 seconds.

- Repeat 10–15 times.

- Repeat 10–15 times with other leg.

- Repeat 10–15 more times with each leg.

Safety Tips

- Have a sturdy chair or a person nearby to hold on to if you feel unsteady.

- Talk with your doctor if you are unsure about doing a particular balance exercise.

Exercising For Flexibility

Flexibility exercises stretch your muscles and can help your body stay limber. Being flexible gives you more freedom of movement for other exercises as well as for your everyday activities.

- Shoulder and upper arm stretch

- Calf stretch

- Yoga

How Much, How Often

Do each stretching exercise 3 to 5 times at each session. Slowly and smoothly stretch into the desired position, as far as possible without pain. Hold the stretch for 10 to 30 seconds. Relax, breathe, then repeat, trying to stretch farther.

Progressing

As you become more flexible, try reaching farther in each exercise. But don't go so far that it hurts.

Exercise Instructions

This exercise to increase flexibility in your shoulders and upper arms will help make it easier to reach for your seatbelt. If you have shoulder problems, talk with your doctor before trying this stretch.

Targeted muscles:

Shoulders and upper arms

What you need:

Towel

- Stand with feet shoulder-width apart.

- Hold one end of a towel in your right hand.

- Raise and bend your right arm to drape the towel down your back. Keep your right arm in this position and continue holding onto the towel.

- Reach behind your lower back and grasp the towel with your left hand.

- To stretch your right shoulder, pull the towel down with your left hand. Stop when you feel a stretch or slight discomfort in your right shoulder.

- Repeat at least 3–5 times.

- Reverse positions, and repeat at least 3–5 times.

Safety Tips

- If you've had hip or back surgery, talk with your doctor before doing lower-back flexibility exercises.

- Always warm-up before stretching exercises. Stretching your muscles before they are warmed up can result in injury. If you are doing only stretching exercises, warm-up with a few minutes of easy walking first. If you are doing endurance or strength exercises, stretch after, not before.

- Always remember to breathe normally while holding a stretch.

- A mild pulling feeling while you are stretching is normal. If you feel sharp or stabbing pain or joint pain, you're stretching too far. Reduce the stretch so it doesn't hurt.

- Always stretch with a smooth, steady movement. Don't jerk or bounce into the stretch; it may cause injury.

- Avoid "locking" your joints. Straighten your arms and legs when you stretch them, but don't hold them tightly in a straight position. Always keep them slightly bent while stretching.

Chapter 18

Cardiovascular (Cardio) Exercise

Cardio Counts

Cardiovascular exercise (also known as aerobic exercise) involves movement that gets your heart rate up to improve how your body uses oxygen. Cardio is considered to be an essential part of any exercise program.

Cardio can help you:

- Strengthen heart and lungs

- Reduce stress and improve mood

- Lower blood pressure

- Lose or maintain weight

- Reduce risk of heart disease and some types of cancer

- Sleep better

- Buildup endurance so you can be active longer

Any amount of cardiovascular exercise has benefits for your health. But different intensities of cardiovascular exercise can be right for different people.

About This Chapter: Text under the heading "Cardio Counts" is excerpted from "Cardio Counts," Smokefree. gov, U.S. Department of Health and Human Services (HHS), January 13, 2017; Text under the heading "Aerobic Activity" is excerpted from "Types Of Physical Activity," National Heart, Lung, and Blood Institute (NHLBI), June 22, 2016; Text under the heading "Types Of Moderate- And Vigorous-Intensity Aerobic Activities" is excerpted from "Physical Activity—Aerobic, Muscle- And Bone-Strengthening: What Counts?" Centers for Disease Control and Prevention (CDC), June 5, 2015.

Moderate-Intensity Activities

Moderate-intensity cardio can be especially good for people starting an exercise program. It raises your heart rate to a point where you sweat and feel you're working. Walking briskly, ballroom dancing, and general gardening are examples of moderate-intensity cardio activities.

High-Intensity Activities

High-intensity cardio can help you burn more calories in less time than a moderate-intensity activity in that same amount of time. Some studies show that vigorous exercise, compared to moderate-intensity exercise, is linked with living longer. Running, swimming laps, and jumping rope are examples of high-intensity cardio. If you have a serious medical condition, are older, or have never done vigorous exercise before, discuss your plan for high-intensity cardio with your doctor before you start.

How Hard Are You Working?

Use the talk test to measure the intensity of your workout. You're doing moderate-intensity activity if you can talk, but not sing. You're doing high-intensity activity if you can say only a few words without pausing for a breath.

Aerobic Activity

Aerobic activity is the type that benefits your heart and lungs the most. Aerobic activity moves your large muscles, such as those in your arms and legs. Running, swimming, walking, bicycling, dancing, and doing jumping jacks are examples of aerobic activity. Aerobic activity also is called endurance activity. Aerobic activity makes your heart beat faster than usual. You also breathe harder during this type of activity. Over time, regular aerobic activity makes your heart and lungs stronger and able to work better.

Levels Of Intensity In Aerobic Activity

You can do aerobic activity with light, moderate, or vigorous intensity. Moderate- and vigorous-intensity aerobic activities are better for your heart than light-intensity activities. However, even light-intensity activities are better than no activity at all. The level of intensity depends on how hard you have to work to do the activity. To do the same activity, people who are less fit usually have to work harder than people who are more fit. So, for example, what is light-intensity activity for one person may be moderate-intensity for another.

Vigorous-Intensity Activities

Vigorous-intensity activities make your heart, lungs, and muscles work hard. On a scale of 0 to 10, vigorous-intensity activity is a 7 or 8. A person doing vigorous-intensity activity can't say more than a few words without stopping for a breath.

Examples Of Aerobic Activities

Below are examples of aerobic activities. Depending on your level of fitness, they can be light, moderate, or vigorous in intensity:

- Pushing a grocery cart around a store
- Gardening, such as digging or hoeing that causes your heart rate to go up
- Walking, hiking, jogging, running
- Water aerobics or swimming laps
- Bicycling, skateboarding, rollerblading, and jumping rope
- Ballroom dancing and aerobic dancing
- Tennis, soccer, hockey, and basketball

People who do moderate- or vigorous-intensity aerobic physical activity have a significantly lower risk of cardiovascular disease than do inactive people. Regularly active people have lower rates of heart disease and stroke, and have lower blood pressure, better blood lipid profiles, and fitness. Significant reductions in risk of cardiovascular disease occur at activity levels equivalent to 150 minutes a week of moderate-intensity physical activity. Even greater benefits are seen with 200 minutes (3 hours and 20 minutes) a week. The evidence is strong that greater amounts of physical activity result in even further reductions in the risk of cardiovascular disease.

(Source: "Chapter 2: Physical Activity Has Many Health Benefits." Office of Disease Prevention and Health Promotion (ODPHP).)

Types Of Moderate- And Vigorous- Intensity Aerobic Activities

Moderate-Intensity Aerobic

For children

- Active recreation such as hiking, skateboarding, rollerblading

- Bicycle riding
- Walking to school

For adolescents

- Active recreation, such as canoeing, hiking, cross-country skiing, skateboarding, rollerblading
- Brisk walking
- Bicycle riding (stationary or road bike)
- House and yard work such as sweeping or pushing a lawn mower
- Playing games that require catching and throwing, such as baseball, softball, basketball and volleyball

Vigorous-Intensity Aerobic

For children

- Active games involving running and chasing, such as tag
- Bicycle riding
- Jumping rope
- Martial arts, such as karate
- Running
- Sports such as ice or field hockey, basketball, swimming, tennis or gymnastics

For adolescents

- Active games involving running and chasing, such as flag football, soccer
- Bicycle riding
- Jumping rope
- Martial arts such as karate
- Running
- Sports such as tennis, ice or field hockey, basketball, swimming
- Vigorous dancing
- Aerobics
- Cheerleading or gymnastics

Chapter 19

Start Running

Take Stock Of Your Current Health And Fitness Level

If you know you have no major health problems, starting a light to moderate intensity exercise program such as brisk walking usually does not require a physical, but check with your doctor for his or her opinion in your specific case. Remember that the health risks of a sedentary lifestyle are much greater than the risks of exercise. A renowned Exercise Physiologist, Per Olaf Astrand, quipped that if one plans a sedentary lifestyle, one should have a physical to see if the heart can stand it!

Be Safe

Don't run/walk in "high crime" areas. When running after dark, be sure to wear reflective clothing, carry a small flashlight, and assume drivers don't see you. Well-lighted neighborhoods are a good choice. Women should run with a partner or a dog if possible, and consider carrying pepper spray. Runners and walkers should never use headphones outdoors, as it makes it impossible to hear traffic or an approaching attacker. Always carry ID.

Start Slowly And Build Up Gradually

Most people should start with a brisk walking program and progress to a mix of alternating walking and jogging. Eventually you should be able to run the entire distance you desire at a

About This Chapter: This chapter includes text excerpted from "Starting A Running Program," U.S. Customs and Border Protection (CBP), January 23, 2014. Reviewed September 2017.

comfortable pace. At that point you can increase weekly mileage about 10% every 3rd week, depending on your goals. For health and fitness there is generally no need to run more than about 15 miles per week, along with some strength and flexibility training. Those wishing to progress to competitive running should seek out experienced runners or coaches for advice.

Using The Right Type Of Shoes Helps Prevent Injuries

Shin splints and runner's knee are preventable with proper conditioning AND the right running shoe type. There are 3 basic types for different running mechanics:

- **Motion Control:** Generally best choice for flat feet and "floppy ankles" (over pronation or rolling too far to the inside after foot touches down). Shoes should be straight lasted and often will have a full board last inside plus a harder rubber or plastic area on the inner (arch support) side of heel to control excess movement.

- **Stability:** Generally best for normal arches, will have a semi-curved last and a moderate amount of motion control.

- **Cushioned:** Generally best for high arches and "clunk foot"; these feet are usually very rigid and 'under pronate," i.e., feet do not roll to the inside far enough after foot touches down and therefore make poor shock absorbers. Shoes should have a curved or semi-curved last, extra cushioning, a full slip last (no board inside), and be very flexible.

Another choice, for off road running are trail running shoes. These are made low to the ground and more stable to help prevent ankle sprains, have good traction, and help prevent foot bruises from roots, rocks, etc.

Don't use any type running shoes for other sports, as they are not made for lateral movements, making ankle sprains more likely. They also last longer and maintain cushioning better if only used for running. Use only good quality court shoes or cross-trainers for other conditioning activities. Wrestling shoes are recommended for defensive tactics training on matted floors.

Do The "Wet Test" To See What Type Of Foot You Have

Wet feet and step onto some paper on a hard surface. (Even better is to run a short distance barefoot on sand.) A "blob" footprint with little arch indicates flat feet. Two 'islands' with a lot of space between the heel and ball indicates high arches. A normal arch will look like the classic cartoon footprint.

Make Sure The Shoe Fits!

The best shoe for you is one that fits your foot type and running mechanics and also is the right length and width. Try on running shoes with the socks you plan to run in, and toward the end of the day when feet are larger. You should have about one thumb's width of room between your longest toe and the end of the shoe. Shoes should be wide enough that foot does not feel pinched on the sides, but not a sloppy fit or one that slips at the heel. Jog a bit in the store to see how the shoes feel and fit. Most running specialty stores such as Fleet Feet in Savannah or 1stPlaceSports in Jacksonville will have the expertise and take the time to fit you properly in several models and watch you run in them before you choose. Don't count on the employees of a general sporting goods or discount footwear store understanding any of the above running shoe information!

Dress For The Weather

In cold weather wear several lightweight layers, hat and gloves to trap body heat. You can unzip or remove layers if you get too warm. In hot weather wear as little as the law allows, and don't forget the sunscreen. Drink plenty of fluids throughout the day to avoid dehydration and plan ahead so you can get fluids during longer runs.

Run With Good Form

Shoulders should be relaxed with elbows bent to about 90 degrees as arms swing smoothly forward and back with no twisting of the torso. Arms should not cross the center of body and hands should pass just above the "hip pocket" on each forward and backward motion. The upper body should be nearly upright, with a very slight forward lean. Don't run on the toes or hit hard with the heel, but rather land as softly as possible with foot nearly flat. The foot should be flexed upward slightly just before foot lands. Breathe naturally through both the nose and mouth. If you're gasping for air slow down!

Most Running Injuries Are Avoidable!

Following the tips on proper footwear, form, and starting slowly will greatly reduce your chances of common beginners' complaints such as shin splints and knee pain. Basic strength and flexibility exercises can prevent and correct muscle imbalances responsible for most running injuries. If you do have a running injury, find the cause rather than just treating the symptoms.

Ignore The Myths

The bulk of scientific evidence shows that running, even in ultra-marathon runners, does not cause osteoarthritis in the hips or knees if these joints were healthy to begin with. In fact, weight-bearing exercise such as running probably prevents arthritis, since the incidence in long-time runners is about half that of nonrunners, including swimmers.

Chapter 20

Calisthenics

Calisthenics are an integral part of a wellrounded physical fitness program because they develop both muscular and aerobic endurance. They are used to warm up and limber the body for sports activities or weight-resistant training and also for cooling down afterward. Calisthenics are low-resistance, high-repetition training.

(Source: "Calisthenics," U.S. Department of Veterans Affairs (VA).)

Physical Fitness

Strong muscles and bones are important to overall health. They are necessary for performing chores and tasks at home, at school, or while playing. When lifting an object off the floor, pushing up out of bed, or bending to see under an object, you use upper and lower body strength. Physical activities such as these will help keep muscles and bones strong!

Fitness Activities And Their Benefits

Muscle fitness can be developed and maintained using calisthenics, free weights, weight machines, or a combination of all three. When developing a muscular strength and muscular

About This Chapter: Text under the heading "Physical Fitness" is excerpted from "Crew Strength Training," National Aeronautics and Space Administration (NASA), July 21, 2012. Reviewed September 2017; Text under the heading "Fitness Activities And Their Benefits" is excerpted from "Muscular Strength And Muscular Endurance," National Interagency Fire Center (NIFC), June 19, 2017; Text beginning with the heading "Some Body Weight Exercise Routines" is excerpted from "Resistance Exercises For Health And Function," Smokefree. gov, U.S. Department of Health and Human Services (HHS), June 16, 2017; Text under the heading "Tips To Follow For Your Strength Training Program" is excerpted from "Train Like An Astronaut: Adapted Physical Activity Strategies," National Aeronautics and Space Administration (NASA), February 24, 2017.

endurance program, it is important to factor in variety in order to maintain interest and utilize the muscles in different ways. Recuperation time between muscle workouts is also important in order to minimize injuries and overuse.

Some of the known benefits of establishing a good fitness program that incorporates muscular strength and endurance activities are as follows:

- Promotes positive changes in bone density

- Promotes positive changes in body composition (increase in lean muscle tissue, decrease in body fat)

- Plays an important role in injury prevention

- Improves sports performance

- Increases lean body mass

- Increases metabolism which can lead to a healthy body weight through the increased caloric use

- Increases the body's balance and coordination

- Maintains the muscle mass needed to burn fat.

Some Body Weight Exercise Routines

Body Weight Squats

- Start sitting at the very edge of a hard chair or bench with your feet hip width apart and your toes just in front of your knees. Cross your arms in front of your chest then raise your elbows to point forward so that your upper arms are parallel to the floor. Make sure you are "tied up" then press through your heels to stand up. DO NOT lock your knees out when you reach the top.

- Leading with your tailbone, sit back down just until your bottom touches the chair and stand right back up. Repeat.

- To add resistance place the resistance band under your feet and, while seated as described above, wrap the extra length around your hand to take up the slack. The band will stretch as you stand. Since your hands will be down to hold the band, be sure to keep your shoulders back and chest out throughout the motion

Push-Ups: There Are 4 Different Ways To Do A Push-Up

1. **Wall Push-Up**

   - Face a wall and raise your arms in front of you up to shoulder level.

   - Place your hands against the wall so they are slightly wider than your shoulders and your fingers are pointing up.

   - Move your feet about 2 feet away from the wall so that your arms are bent as you lean into the wall on an angle. Be sure you are "tied up" so that your back stays flat like in the plank exercise.

   - Now, push your upper body away from the wall until your arms are extended (DO NOT LOCK elbows).

   - Repeat.

2. **Incline Push-Up**

   - Stand facing a bench or sturdy elevated platform.

   - Place hands on the edge, slightly wider than your shoulders.

   - Move your feet back far enough to ensure that your arms are at 90° to your body and your back is straight (like the plank). You will be on the balls of your feet.

   - Now, lower your chest to the edge of the platform by bending your elbows. Push your body back into the starting position until arms are extended (Do NOT LOCK elbows).

   - Repeat.

3. **Modified Push-Up**

   - The best way to get into the modified position is to start in the full position. This is basically the plank on your hands instead of your forearms.

   - Now, from this position simply drop your knees to the floor and lift and cross your feet. Your body should still be stretched out and your back should be flat. (No sagging backs or bottoms up in the air!)

   - Lower your chest to the floor by bending your elbows to about 90 degrees (This is when your bottom wants to stay in the air!) Be sure to keep your back flat. Now, push yourself back to the starting position. (This is when a sagging back is likely to happen!) Be sure to keep your back flat like the plank.

   - Repeat.

4. Full Push-Up

- The starting position for this push-up is basically the plank on your hands instead of your forearms and up on your toes.

- Lower your chest to the floor by bending your elbows to about 90 degrees (This is when your bottom wants to stay in the air!) Be sure to keep your back flat.

- Now, push yourself back to the starting position. (This is when a sagging back is likely to happen!) Be sure to keep your back flat like the plank.

- Repeat.

Wall Sits

- Start with your back up against a smooth wall.

- Place your feet hip width apart about 1–1 ½ feet away from the wall.

- Slide your back down the wall until your thighs are parallel to the floor. Be sure your knees do not extend past your toes. If they do, move your feet further from the wall.

- Hold the sit for a long as you are able then push up through you heels to slide your back up the wall.

- Rest and repeat.

Standing Lunges

- Start with your feet together then take a large step forward with one foot. Your rear foot should be on its toes.

- Stand with nice upright posture and place your hands on your hip. Now, slowly lower your rear knee straight down to the floor until your front knee is at 90 degrees (Your knee should not pass your toes).

- Press up to return to the starting position being sure to maintain your upright posture.

- Repeat with the opposite foot in front.

- To add resistance you can hold dumbbells at your sides.

Calf Raises

- Start with your feet flat on the floor.

- Raise yourself up onto your toes, pause, and slowly lower yourself back to the starting position.

- Repeat. Hint, if you are having trouble balancing, hold on to something sturdy like a countertop or the back of a sturdy chair. Make sure you are "tied up"… it helps with balance!

Curl-Ups

- Start by lying on your back with knees bent and feet flat on the floor.

- Place your hands either by your ears or across your chest. Make sure you are "tied up" and slowly curl up until your shoulder blades are just off the floor. This is NOT a full sit-up! Picture a string attached to your chest pulling through your belly button. You should feel it in your abs NOT your neck!

Front Planks

- Start by lying face down. Place your elbows and forearms under your chest.

- Using your toes and forearms, prop yourself up to form a bridge. Maintain a flat back and do not allow your bottom to stick up into the air or your back to sag.

- Hold this position for 10 seconds to start and gradually increase the length of the hold. Keep your abs tight ("tie it up").

- Rest and repeat.

TRY THIS! Some Ideas For Adapted Activity

Push-Ups And/Or Related Exercises

- Perform at various levels: table, stool, bench, wall or wall bar, steps, etc.

- Wheelchair push up: Seated in chair with arms, place hands on arm rests and lift body. Hold position In push up position, alternate right and left hand crossing midline to touch opposite shoulder, keeping plank; attempt in wall push up position.

Plank And/Or Related Exercises

- Perform at various levels: table, stool, bench, wall or wall bar, steps, etc.

- While in plank, place ball between body and floor and use hands, walk out and back.

Seated Isometric Exercises

- In a chair or at bench edge, hold, breathe, and squeeze abdominal muscles Wall sit with back against wall, knees @ 90 degrees; hold, breathe, and squeeze abdominal muscles.

- On a core ball, knees @ 90 degrees; squeeze abdominal muscles.

Tips To Follow For Your Strength Training Program

Warm up for 5–10 minutes. This will reduce your chance of getting hurt and increase your range of motion. Use your walk as a warm-up or walk in place for a few minutes. Do a few stretches for the muscles you will be working on that day.

Follow the instructions for the exercises carefully. Some of the old ways you may have learned to train your muscles may not be as safe or effective. (For example: You may have been taught to do sit-ups with your legs straight out. Now it's known that it's important to bend your knees to prevent back problems.)

After you exercise muscles on one side of a joint, exercise those on the other side. This helps to maintain balance and prevent injury. (For example: If you first exercise the muscles that bend the elbow (biceps) then exercise the muscles that straighten the elbow (triceps).

Move slowly and smoothly. Never hold your breath.

- When you lift: Breathe out, and count 1–2.

- Hold the position for 1 count.

- When you release: Breathe in and count 1-2-3-4. Be careful to control the speed with which you release the movement. This will avoid stressing the joints.

Do each exercise through the full range of motion. If you can't do this, decrease the amount of resistance.

Keep it slow and steady

- Add more resistance gradually to develop muscle strength. But also be careful not to do too much.

- You may want to slowly repeat each exercise 10–20 times (this is called a "set"). Then work up to doing 2–3 sets of each exercise each time.

- When using the exercise bands, it's okay to do the exercises every day unless you use too much resistance and your muscles are very sore. If you are very sore it is best to take a day off to allow your muscles to rest and recover. Always cool down after the exercises by stretching the muscle groups used.

Chapter 21

Strength Training

To do most of the strength exercises, you will need to lift or push weights (or your own body weight), and gradually increase the amount of weight used. Dumbbells and hand/ankle weights sold in sporting goods stores as well as resistance tubing can be purchased. Get creative and use things in your home like milk or water jugs filled with sand or water, or socks filled with beans and tied shut at the ends. You can also use the special strength training equipment at a gym or fitness center. There are so many ways to participate in strength training!

Strength training activities include:

- Using your own body (e.g., push-ups, squats, etc.)
- Using resistance bands
- Using weights or things around the house (like soup cans) for exercises like bicep curls
- Using weight equipment at a gym like a leg curl machine

(Source: "What Are Strength Training Activities?" Smokefree.gov, U.S. Department of Health and Human Services (HHS).)

How Much, How Often

- Do strength exercises for all of your major muscle groups at least twice a week, but no more than 3 times per week.

About This Chapter: This chapter includes text excerpted from "Sample Strength Activity Plan For Beginners," U.S. Department of Veterans Affairs (VA), March 13, 2014. Reviewed September 2017.

- Don't do strength exercises of the same muscle group on any 2 days in a row.

- Depending on your condition, you might need to start out using 1 or 2 pounds of weight or no weight at all. Sometimes, the weight of your arms or legs alone is enough to get you started.

- Use a minimum weight the first week, and then gradually add weight. Starting out with weights that are too heavy can cause injuries.

- Gradually add a challenging amount of weight to your strength routine. If you don't challenge your muscles, you won't get much benefit.

How To Do Strength Exercises

- Do 8–12 repetitions in a row. Wait a minute, and then do another "set" of 8–12 repetitions of the same exercise.

- Take 3 seconds to lift or push a weight into place; hold the position for 1 second, and take another 3 seconds to lower the weight. Don't let the weight drop or let your arms or legs fall in an uncontrolled way. Lowering slowly is very important.

- It should feel somewhere between hard and very hard (15–17 on the Borg Scale) for you to lift or push the weight. It should not feel very, very hard. If you can't lift or push at least 8 times in a row, it's too heavy for you. Reduce the amount of weight. If you can lift more than 12 times in a row without much difficulty, then it's too light for you. Try increasing the amount of weight you are lifting. A little extra weight goes a long way!

- Stretch after strength exercises, as this is when your muscles are warmed up. If you stretch before strength exercises, be sure to warm up your muscles first by light walking and arm pumping.

Safety

- Don't hold your breath or strain during strength exercises. Breathe out as you lift or push, and breathe in as you relax; this may not feel natural at first. Counting out loud helps.

- If you have had your hip or knee joint replaced, check with your doctor to see if there are some lower body exercises that you should skip.

- Avoid jerking or thrusting weights into position or "locking" the joints in your arms and legs. This can cause injuries. Use smooth, steady movements.

- Muscle soreness lasting up to a few days and slight fatigue are normal after muscle-building exercises. Exhaustion, sore joints, and unpleasant muscle pulling are not. These problems mean you are overdoing it.

- None of the exercises should cause pain.

Progressing

- Gradually increasing the amount of weight you use is crucial for building strength.

- When you are able to lift a weight more than 12 times, increase the amount of weight you use at your next session.

- Here is an example of how to progress gradually:

- Start out with a weight that you can lift only 8 times.

- Keep using that weight until you become strong enough to lift it 12 to 15 times.

- Add more weight so that, again, you can lift it only 8 times.

- Use this weight until you can lift it 12 to 15 times, and then add more weight. Keep repeating.

Examples Of Strength Exercises

Arm Raise

Strengthens shoulder muscles.

- Sit in armless chair with your back supported by back of chair.

- Keep feet flat on floor even with your shoulders.

- Hold hand weights straight down at your sides, with palms facing inward.

- Raise both arms to side, shoulder height.

- Hold the position for 1 second.

- Slowly lower arms to sides. Pause.

- Repeat 8 to 12 times.

- Rest, then do another set of 8 to 12 repetitions.

Chair Stand

Strengthens muscles in abdomen and thighs. Your goal is to do this exercise without using your hands as you become stronger.

- Place pillows on the back of chair.

- Sit toward front of chair, knees bent, feet flat on floor.

- Lean back on pillows in half-reclining position. Keep your back and shoulders straight throughout exercise.

- Raise upper body forward until sitting upright, using hands as little as possible (or not at all, if you can). Your back should no longer lean against pillows.

- Slowly stand up, using hands as little as possible.

- Slowly sit back down. Pause.

- Repeat 8 to 12 times.

- Rest, then do another set of 8 to 12 repetitions.

Biceps Curl

Strengthens upper-arm muscles.

- Sit in armless chair with your back supported by back of chair.

- Keep feet flat on floor even with your shoulders.

- Hold hand weights straight down at your sides, with palms facing inward.

- Slowly bend one elbow, lifting weight toward chest. (Rotate palm to face shoulder while lifting weight.)

- Hold position for 1 second.

- Slowly lower arm to starting position. Pause.

- Repeat with other arm.

- Alternate arms until you have done 8 to 12 repetitions with each arm.

- Rest, then do another set of 8 to 12 alternating repetitions.

Plantar Flexion

Strengthens ankle and calf muscles. Use ankle weights if you are ready.

- Stand straight, feet flat on floor, holding onto a table or chair for balance.
- Slowly stand on tiptoe, as high as possible.
- Hold position for 1 second.
- Slowly lower heels all the way back down. Pause.
- Do the exercise 8 to 12 times.
- Rest, then do another set of 8 to 12 repetitions.

Variation:

As you become stronger, do the exercise standing on one leg only, alternating legs for a total of 8 to 12 times on each leg. Rest, then do another set of 8 to 12 alternating repetitions.

Triceps Extension

Strengthens muscles in back of upper arm. Keep supporting your arm with your hand throughout the exercise. (If your shoulders aren't flexible enough to do this exercise, focus on shoulder stretching exercises.)

- Sit in chair with your back supported by back of chair.
- Keep feet flat on floor even with shoulders.
- Hold a weight in one hand. Raise that arm straight toward ceiling, palm facing in.
- Support this arm, below elbow, with other hand.
- Slowly bend raised arm at elbow, bringing hand weight toward same shoulder.
- Slowly straighten arm toward ceiling.
- Hold position for 1 second.
- Slowly bend arm toward shoulder again. Pause.
- Repeat the bending and straightening until you have done the exercise 8 to 12 times.
- Repeat 8 to 12 times with your other arm.
- Rest, then do another set of 8 to 12 alternating repetitions.

Knee Flexion

Strengthens muscles in back of thigh. Use ankle weights if you are ready.

- Stand straight holding onto a table or chair for balance.

- Slowly bend knee as far as possible. Don't move your upper leg at all; bend your knee only.

- Hold position for 1 second.

- Slowly lower foot all the way back down. Pause.

- Repeat with other leg.

- Alternate legs until you have done 8 to 12 repetitions with each leg.

- Rest, then do another set of 8 to 12 alternating repetitions.

Hip Flexion

Strengthens thigh and hip muscles. Use ankle weights, if you are ready.

- Stand straight to the side or behind a chair or table, holding on for balance.

- Slowly bend one knee toward chest, without bending waist or hips.

- Hold position for 1 second.

- Slowly lower leg all the way down. Pause.

- Repeat with other leg.

- Alternate legs until you have done 8 to 12 repetitions with each leg.

- Rest, then do another set of 8 to 12 alternating repetitions.

Shoulder Flexion

Strengthens shoulder muscles.

- Sit in armless chair with your back supported by back of chair.

- Keep feet flat on floor even with your shoulders.

- Hold hand weights straight down at your sides, with palms facing inward.

- Raise both arms in front of you (keep them straight and rotate so palms face downward) to shoulder height.

- Hold position for 1 second.

- Slowly lower arms to sides. Pause.

- Repeat 8 to 12 times.

- Rest, then do another set of 8 to 12 repetitions.

Knee Extension

Strengthens muscles in front of thigh and shin. Use ankle weights if you are ready.

- Sit in chair. Only the balls of your feet and your toes should rest on the floor. Put rolled towel under knees, if needed, to lift your feet. Rest your hands on your thighs or on the sides of the chair.
- Slowly extend one leg in front of you as straight as possible.
- Flex ankle so that toes are pulled back towards head.
- Hold position for 1 to 2 seconds.
- Slowly lower leg back down. Pause.
- Repeat with other leg.
- Alternate legs until you have done 8 to 12 repetitions with each leg.
- Rest, then do another set of 8 to 12 alternating repetitions.

Hip Extension

Strengthens buttock and lower-back muscles. Use ankle weights, if you are ready.

- Stand 12 to 18 inches from a table or chair, feet slightly apart.
- Bend forward at hips at about 45-degree angle; hold onto a table or chair for balance.
- Slowly lift one leg straight backwards without bending your knee, pointing your toes, or bending your upper body any farther forward.
- Hold position for 1 second.
- Slowly lower leg. Pause.
- Repeat with other leg.
- Alternate legs until you have done 8 to 12 repetitions with each leg.
- Rest, then do another set of 8 to 12 alternating repetitions.

Side Leg Raise

Strengthens muscles at sides of hips and thighs. Use ankle weights, if you are ready.

- Stand straight, directly behind table or chair, feet slightly apart.

- Hold onto a table or chair for balance.

- Slowly lift one leg 6–12 inches out to side. Keep your back and both legs straight. Don't point your toes outward; keep them facing forward.

- Hold position for 1 second.

- Slowly lower leg. Pause.

- Repeat with other leg.

- Alternate legs until you have done 8 to 12 repetitions with each leg.

- Rest, then do another set of 8 to 12 alternating repetitions.

Chapter 22

Stretching

Ways To Stretch

Stretching can help make you more flexible, so you can do activities more easily. It also lengthens and loosens tight muscles.

Stretches To Try

1. **Cross shoulder stretch**

   Sit or stand up straight. Keep shoulders even. Extend right arm across chest. Place left hand on the right elbow to gently support your arm. Feel the stretch in your right arm and shoulder. Breathe in through your nose, and breathe out through your mouth. Hold stretch for a count of 15. Repeat this stretch on opposite side, using right hand to stretch left arm and shoulder.

2. **Triceps stretch**

   Stand up straight, with knees slightly bent, toes facing forward. Place feet hip distance apart. Keep shoulders even. Bend right arm at elbow, with elbow pointing to the sky. Lift arm next to your head. Position right fingers so they touch the shoulder blade area. Place left arm across top of head, and place left hand on the right elbow to gently support the arm during this stretch. You should feel a stretch in the back of your right arm. Breathe in through your nose, and breathe out through your mouth.

About This Chapter: This chapter includes text excerpted from "Ways To Stretch," girlshealth.gov, Office on Women's Health (OWH), March 27, 2015.

Hold stretch for a count of 15. Repeat this stretch on the opposite side, using right hand to stretch left triceps.

3. **Chest stretch**

Stand up straight, with knees slightly bent, toes facing forward. Place feet hip distance apart. Keep shoulders even. Place arms behind your back. Clasp your hands together, lifting your arms behind your back. Squeeze your shoulder blades together. Feel the stretch in your chest. Breathe in through your nose, and breathe out through your mouth. Hold stretch for count of 15.

4. **Quadriceps stretch**

You're going to be standing on one leg, so you may want help staying steady. If so, stand facing a wall or other surface, about 1 foot away from it. Put your right hand against the wall. Raise your left leg behind you and gently grab your foot with your left hand. Relax your left foot in your hand. Press your right hip forward to stretch the muscles in the front of your left thigh. Keep your knees close together. Hold stretch for a count of 15. Repeat the stretch with your right leg.

5. **Hamstring stretch**

Lie with your back flat on the floor, with both of your knees bent. Place your feet flat on the floor, about 6 inches apart. Straighten your right knee and put both hands behind your right knee. Slowly lift your right leg, feeling a slight stretching in the back of your thigh. Keep your head relaxed on the floor. If you cannot relax your head on the floor, place a towel around your calf or ankle, holding one side of the towel in each hand. Hold stretch for a count of 15. Repeat the stretch with your left leg.

6. **Runner's stretch**

Squat down and put both hands on the floor in front of you. Stretch your right leg straight out behind you and relax your knee on the ground. Keep your left foot flat on the floor and lean forward with your chest on your left knee. Move your weight back to your right leg, keeping it as straight as you can. Do not move your left knee farther forward than your left ankle. Hold stretch for a count of 15. Repeat the stretch with your left leg.

7. **Calf stretch**

Stand facing a wall or other surface, about 2 feet away from it, keeping your heels flat and your back straight. Lean forward and press your hands against the wall. Take one step forward with your left leg and bend the knee slightly. Keep your right leg straight and your heel on the ground. Stand up tall with shoulders over hips. Make sure your knee does not move in front of your ankle. You should feel stretching in the muscles in the back of your lower right leg, above your heel. If you need a bigger stretch, move your back farther away from the wall. Hold stretch for a count of 15. Repeat the stretch with your left leg.

Stretching Tips

It's a good idea to stretch any time you work out, but try for at least two or three days each week. To stretch well, try these tips:

- **Warm up before you stretch.** Stretching is more helpful when your muscles are warmed up. You can do some light exercises like walking or jogging in place for five to 10 minutes to warm up.

- **Stretch for around 10 minutes.** You can stretch right after you warm up or at the end of your workout—or do both!

- **Go easy on yourself.** You will feel a gentle pull, but if it hurts, stop. And don't forget to breathe.

- **Don't bounce.** A stretch works well if you just hold it. If you are just starting out, try holding a **stretch for around 15 seconds.** If you are more flexible, you can hold it for a minute.

- **Make sure to repeat each stretch on both sides.** Do each stretch two to four times on each side.

Chapter 23

Pilates

What Is Pilates?

Pilates is a fitness regimen for building flexibility, strength, endurance, and coordination. The emphasis is on improving core strength and fitness without adding muscle bulk. Pilates involves controlled movements done on a mat or with equipment. It improves physical and mental well-being, strengthens muscles, and tones the body, while also strengthening the torso and providing better posture and good health. Pilates strongly emphasizes technique, and despite outward appearances it is not as easy as doing crunches or other core-strengthening exercises. The moves look simple, but execution requires precision and control. The exercises have names such as "The 100," "The Elephant," and "The Swan" and are usually done in a specific order, one after the other.

The method was developed by Joseph H. Pilates, a German bodybuilder, gymnast, and physical trainer, who overcame childhood disease and fragility to become an accomplished athlete in various sports. Working as a nurse in Great Britain during World War I, he designed equipment and a system of exercises for rehabilitating immobilized soldiers and other patients. After immigrating to the United States in the 1920s, Pilates taught these exercises in a studio in New York.

What Are The Types Of Pilates Exercises?

Pilates exercises can be generally categorized into two types:

1. The first requires primarily just a floor mat and a training routine and is designed to use body weight for resistance. Of the 500 exercises that were originally developed for

"Pilates," © 2018 Omnigraphics. Reviewed September 2017.

Pilates, 34 are mat-based movements. In addition to the mat, these exercises utilize other traditional Pilates equipment, such as magic circles and hand weights, or non-standard gear like gym balls, stretch bands, and foam rollers.

2. The second type employs specialized equipment, such as "Reformer," "Cadillac," "Wunda Chair," "Spine Corrector," and "Ladder Barrel," which were designed by Pilates himself. This equipment uses a system of pulleys, springs, handles, and straps to provide resistance or support based on the requirements of the exercise.

Both kinds of exercises can be adapted for varying degrees of fitness and ability. If exercising on the mat turns out to be difficult for some people, the equipment offers alternative ways to exercise.

How Does Pilates Work?

Pilates can be practiced with a mat at home—possibly with the guidance of a home video—at a gymnasium or studio with special equipment, or at a class with a trainer. Typically, classes last for 45 minutes to an hour. Pilates, which can be practiced for a few days per week along with aerobics, is considered a medium-intensity regimen, and though you will not necessarily work up a sweat, your muscles will get a thorough workout. Pilates focuses on concentration and breathing, as well as strengthening the core of the body, arms, and legs. It can also improve flexibility and joint mobility while strengthening the muscles and helping maintain a healthy body weight.

Who Can Do Pilates?

Pilates is suitable for people of all ages and fitness levels, from beginners to athletes. The equipment can be calibrated for support, to help beginners and people with health conditions, or for resistance in the case of athletes who want to challenge themselves. As with any exercise routine, it's a good idea to consult a healthcare professional if you have an injury or a medical condition before you begin working out.

What Are The Health Benefits Of Pilates?

The benefits of Pilates can include improved posture, balance, muscle tone, joint mobility, and relief from stress and tension. Pilates has been shown to be particularly beneficial for athletes and dancers, because it helps develop overall body strength and flexibility and reduces the risk of injury. While there is scientific evidence to support many of these benefits, there has not been enough rigorous scrutiny for definitive conclusions. More standardized research in this area is needed in order to verify the benefits scientifically.

What Are The Benefits Of Pilates For People With Health Conditions?

Pilates has the advantage of being adaptable to a variety of individual needs. In many cases, it has been a useful addition to aerobics for people with heart disease, hypertension, and high cholesterol. For people with arthritis, it can be a beneficial strength-training program. Pilates may also be a good choice for lower back pain, helping to strengthen the muscles that support the back. Pregnant women who are already working out with Pilates should be able to continue, with their doctor's approval, as long as modifications are made to accommodate the pregnancy. It is important to understand that people with any medical condition should participate in a Pilates program only after consultation with a healthcare professional.

How Is Pilates Different From Yoga?

Pilates and yoga are different methods of exercises, but both offer similar benefits, such as improved posture, strength, balance, flexibility, and good breathing techniques. Although both systems promote physical and mental health, yoga tends to focus more on meditation and relaxation. Pilates makes use of equipment but yoga does not, and Pilates uses flow of movement, while yoga features static poses.

How Should You Choose A Pilates Class?

Pilates classes are often taught in a studio with equipment or in open areas with mats, and they usually last for about an hour. Ideally, equipment-based Pilates should be taught on a one-to-one basis and mat exercises in small groups to ensure personal attention. If you are joining a group class for equipment training, make sure you gain sufficient familiarity with the equipment before attempting to use it on your own. There are no legal requirements or qualifications needed to become a Pilates instructor. As a result, it's important to choose a teacher or class leader based on experience, recommendations, and personal rapport. Good instructors should have up to 450 hours of experience over a span of several years.

References

1. "A Guide To Pilates," NHS Choices, May 18, 2015.

2. "Pilates," The Nemours Foundation, February 2014.

3. Robinson, Kara Mayer. "Pilates," WebMD, 2017.

Chapter 24

Yoga

Yoga is a mind and body practice with historical origins in ancient Indian philosophy. Like other meditative movement practices used for health purposes, various styles of yoga typically combine physical postures, breathing techniques, and meditation or relaxation. This chapter provides basic information about yoga, summarizes scientific research on effectiveness and safety.

> Yoga in its full form combines physical postures, breathing exercises, meditation, and a distinct philosophy. There are numerous styles of yoga. Hatha yoga, commonly practiced in the United States and Europe, emphasizes postures, breathing exercises, and meditation. Hatha yoga styles include Ananda, Anusara, Ashtanga, Bikram, Iyengar, Kripalu, Kundalini, Viniyoga, and others.

Key Facts

- Studies in people with chronic low-back pain suggest that a carefully adapted set of yoga poses may help reduce pain and improve function (the ability to walk and move). Studies also suggest that practicing yoga (as well as other forms of regular exercise) might have other health benefits such as reducing heart rate and blood pressure, and may also help relieve anxiety and depression. Other research suggests yoga is not helpful for asthma, and studies looking at yoga and arthritis have had mixed results.

About This Chapter: This chapter includes text excerpted from "Yoga: In Depth," National Center for Complementary and Alternative Medicine (NCCAM), National Center for Complementary and Integrative Health (NCCIH), June 2013. Reviewed September 2017.

- People with high blood pressure, glaucoma, or sciatica, and women who are pregnant should modify or avoid some yoga poses.

- Ask a trusted source (such as a healthcare provider or local hospital) to recommend a yoga practitioner. Contact professional organizations for the names of practitioners who have completed an acceptable training program.

- Tell all your healthcare providers about any complementary health approaches you use. Give them a full picture of what you do to manage your health. This will help ensure coordinated and safe care.

What The Science Says About Yoga

Researchers suggest that a carefully adapted set of yoga poses may reduce low-back pain and improve function. Other studies also suggest that practicing yoga (as well as other forms of regular exercise) might improve quality of life; reduce stress; lower heart rate and blood pressure; help relieve anxiety, depression, and insomnia; and improve overall physical fitness, strength, and flexibility. But some research suggests yoga may not improve asthma, and studies looking at yoga and arthritis have had mixed results.

- One NCCIH-funded study of 90 people with chronic low-back pain found that participants who practiced Iyengar yoga had significantly less disability, pain, and depression after 6 months.

- In another study, also funded by NCCIH, researchers compared yoga with conventional stretching exercises or a selfcare book in 228 adults with chronic low-back pain. The results showed that both yoga and stretching were more effective than a selfcare book for improving function and reducing symptoms due to chronic low-back pain.

- Conclusions from another study of 313 adults with chronic or recurring low-back pain suggested that 12 weekly yoga classes resulted in better function than usual medical care.

However, studies show that certain health conditions may not benefit from yoga.

- A systematic review of clinical studies suggests that there is no sound evidence that yoga improves asthma.

- A review of the literature reports that few published studies have looked at yoga and arthritis, and of those that have, results are inconclusive. The two main types of arthritis—osteoarthritis and rheumatoid arthritis—are different conditions, and the effects of yoga may not be the same for each. In addition, the reviewers suggested that even if a study showed that yoga helped osteoarthritic finger joints, it may not help osteoarthritic knee joints.

Side Effects And Risks

Yoga is generally low-impact and safe for healthy people when practiced appropriately under the guidance of a well-trained instructor. Overall, those who practice yoga have a low rate of side effects, and the risk of serious injury from yoga is quite low. However, certain types of stroke as well as pain from nerve damage are among the rare possible side effects of practicing yoga. Women who are pregnant and people with certain medical conditions, such as high blood pressure, glaucoma (a condition in which fluid pressure within the eye slowly increases and may damage the eye's optic nerve), and sciatica (pain, weakness, numbing, or tingling that may extend from the lower back to the calf, foot, or even the toes), should modify or avoid some yoga poses.

Training, Licensing, And Certification

There are many training programs for yoga teachers throughout the country. These programs range from a few days to more than 2 years. Standards for teacher training and certification differ depending on the style of yoga.

There are organizations that register yoga teachers and training programs that have complied with a certain curriculum and educational standards. For example, one nonprofit group (the Yoga Alliance) requires at least 200 hours of training, with a specified number of hours in areas including techniques, teaching methodology, anatomy, physiology, and philosophy. Most yoga therapist training programs involve 500 hours or more. The International Association of Yoga Therapists (IAYT) is developing standards for yoga therapy training.

If You Are Considering Practicing Yoga

- Do not use yoga to replace conventional medical care or to postpone seeing a healthcare provider about pain or any other medical condition.

- If you have a medical condition, talk to your healthcare provider before starting yoga.

- Ask a trusted source (such as your healthcare provider or a nearby hospital) to recommend a yoga practitioner. Find out about the training and experience of any practitioner you are considering.

- Everyone's body is different, and yoga postures should be modified based on individual abilities. Carefully selecting an instructor who is experienced with and attentive to your needs is an important step toward helping you practice yoga safely. Ask about the physical demands of the type of yoga in which you are interested and inform your yoga instructor about any medical issues you have.

- Carefully think about the type of yoga you are interested in. For example, hot yoga (such as Bikram yoga) may involve standing and moving in humid environments with temperatures as high as 105°F. Because such settings may be physically stressful, people who practice hot yoga should take certain precautions. These include drinking water before, during, and after a hot yoga practice and wearing suitable clothing. People with conditions that may be affected by excessive heat, such as heart disease, lung disease, and a prior history of heatstroke may want to avoid this form of yoga. Women who are pregnant may want to check with their healthcare providers before starting hot yoga.

- Tell all your healthcare providers about any complementary health approaches you use. Give them a full picture of what you do to manage your health. This will help ensure coordinated and safe care.

Chapter 25

Measuring Exercise Intensity

Relative And Absolute Intensity

Here are some ways to understand and measure the intensity of aerobic activity: relative intensity and absolute intensity.

Relative Intensity

The level of effort required by a person to do an activity. When using relative intensity, people pay attention to how physical activity affects their heart rate and breathing.

The talk test is a simple way to measure relative intensity. In general, if you're doing moderate-intensity activity you can talk, but not sing, during the activity. If you're doing vigorous-intensity activity, you will not be able to say more than a few words without pausing for a breath.

Absolute Intensity

The amount of energy used by the body per minute of activity. Below lists examples of activities classified as moderate-intensity or vigorous-intensity based upon the amount of energy used by the body while doing the activity.

Moderate Intensity

- Walking briskly (3 miles per hour or faster, but not race-walking)

- Water aerobics

About This Chapter: This chapter includes text excerpted from "Physical Activity Basics—Measuring Physical Activity Intensity," Centers for Disease Control and Prevention (CDC), June 4, 2015.

- Bicycling slower than 10 miles per hour

- Tennis (doubles)

- Ballroom dancing

- General gardening

Vigorous Intensity

- Race walking, jogging, or running

- Swimming laps

- Tennis (singles)

- Aerobic dancing

- Bicycling 10 miles per hour or faster

- Jumping rope

- Heavy gardening (continuous digging or hoeing)

- Hiking uphill or with a heavy backpack

Target Heart Rate And Estimated Maximum Heart Rate

One way of monitoring physical activity intensity is to determine whether a person's pulse or heart rate is within the target zone during physical activity.

For moderate-intensity physical activity, a person's target heart rate should be 50 to 70 percent of his or her maximum heart rate. This maximum rate is based on the person's age. An estimate of a person's maximum age-related heart rate can be obtained by subtracting the person's age from 220. For example, for a 50-year-old person, the estimated maximum age-related heart rate would be calculated as 220 - 50 years = 170 beats per minute (bpm). The 50 percent and 70 percent levels would be:

- 50 percent level: 170 x 0.50 = 85 bpm, and

- 70 percent level: 170 x 0.70 = 119 bpm

Thus, moderate-intensity physical activity for a 50-year-old person will require that the heart rate remains between 85 and 119 bpm during physical activity.

For vigorous-intensity physical activity, a person's target heart rate should be 70 to 85 percent of his or her maximum heart rate. To calculate this range, follow the same formula as used above, except change "50 and 70 percent" to "70 and 85 percent." For example, for a 35-year-old person, the estimated maximum age-related heart rate would be calculated as 220 - 35 years = 185 beats per minute (bpm). The 70 percent and 85 percent levels would be:

- 70 percent level: 185 x 0.70 = 130 bpm, and

- 85 percent level: 185 x 0.85 = 157 bpm

Thus, vigorous-intensity physical activity for a 35-year-old person will require that the heart rate remains between 130 and 157 bpm during physical activity.

Taking Your Heart Rate

Generally, to determine whether you are exercising within the heart rate target zone, you must stop exercising briefly to take your pulse. You can take the pulse at the neck, the wrist, or the chest. You can feel the radial pulse on the artery of the wrist in line with the thumb. Place the tips of the index and middle fingers over the artery and press lightly. Do not use the thumb. Take a full 60-second count of the heartbeats, or take for 30 seconds and multiply by 2. Start the count on a beat, which is counted as "zero." If this number falls between 85 and 119 bpm in a person, he or she is active within the target range for moderate-intensity activity.

Perceived Exertion (Borg Rating Of Perceived Exertion Scale)

The Borg Rating of Perceived Exertion (RPE) is a way of measuring physical activity intensity level. Perceived exertion is how hard you feel like your body is working. It is based on the physical sensations a person experiences during physical activity, including increased heart rate, increased respiration or breathing rate, increased sweating, and muscle fatigue. Although this is a subjective measure, a person's exertion rating may provide a fairly good estimate of the actual heart rate during physical activity.

Practitioners generally agree that perceived exertion ratings between 12 to 14 on the Borg Scale suggests that physical activity is being performed at a moderate level of intensity. During activity, use the Borg Scale to assign numbers to how you feel. Self-monitoring how hard your body is working can help you adjust the intensity of the activity by speeding up or slowing down your movements.

Through experience of monitoring how your body feels, it will become easier to know when to adjust your intensity. For example, a walker who wants to engage in moderate-intensity activity would aim for a Borg Scale level of "somewhat hard" (12–14). If he describes his muscle fatigue and breathing as "very light" (9 on the Borg Scale) he would want to increase his intensity. On the other hand, if he felt his exertion was "extremely hard" (19 on the Borg Scale) he would need to slow down his movements to achieve the moderate-intensity range.

A high correlation exists between a person's perceived exertion rating times 10 and the actual heart rate during physical activity; so a person's exertion rating may provide a fairly good estimate of the actual heart rate during activity. For example, if a person's rating of perceived exertion is 12, then 12 x 10 = 120; so the heart rate should be approximately 120 beats per minute. Note that this calculation is only an approximation of heart rate, and the actual heart rate can vary quite a bit depending on age and physical condition. The Borg Rating of Perceived Exertion is also the preferred method to assess intensity among those individuals who take medications that affect heart rate or pulse.

Part Four
Activities For Team Athletes And Individuals

Chapter 26

Choosing The Right Sport For You

Why Choose Sports?

Playing sports can help you make friends, boost your mood, and teach you tons of skills. Teens who play sports may:

- Have greater self-esteem and less depression

- Learn how to set goals and work hard

- Have a more positive body image

- Learn about working as part of a team

- Do better in school

Picking A Sport

It helps to think about a few issues when choosing a sport. Start by asking yourself some questions:

- Do you like to work together with teammates, the way you do in soccer or lacrosse?

- Do you prefer to work more on your own, as in swimming or track?

- How do you feel about competition? Does it twist your tummy? Maybe inviting a friend to shoot hoops or go hiking is more for you.

- Do you like to keep moving? Does soccer, basketball, or field hockey sound fun to you?

About This Chapter: This chapter includes text excerpted from "Playing Sports," girlshealth.gov, Office on Women's Health (OWH), March 27, 2015.

- Do you like music? You might think about dance and cheerleading, which can offer great workouts.

- Are you interested in relaxing and connecting your mind and body, like you do in yoga or Pilates?

Few sports and activities include:

- Ballet
- Baseball
- Basketball
- Bicycling
- Canoeing/kayaking
- Cheerleading
- Diving
- Figure Skating
- Fishing
- Football
- Frisbee
- Golf
- Gymnastics
- Hiking
- Horseback Riding
- Inline Skating

- Jump Rope
- Martial Arts
- Skateboarding
- Snorkeling
- Snow Skiing
- Soccer
- Softball
- Surfing
- Swimming
- Table Tennis
- Tennis
- Volleyball
- Walking
- White-Water Rafting
- Yoga

Team Time

Are you on a team? That's great. Playing on a team can offer amazing benefits—and fun. But you may need to spend time being active in addition to your team practices. Experts say that many players don't get the recommended "dose" of daily exercise during practice. Remember, your body needs 60 minutes of activity every day (and time on the bench doesn't count)!

Safety In Sports

Stay in the game with these tips:

- **If you're new to a sport,** work your way up slowly.

- **Before you start a sport, see your doctor for a sports physical.** Some states require these examinations to make sure you are healthy enough to play. But even if a sports physical is not required, it makes good sense to get one.

- **Follow safety rules for your sport.** In cheerleading, for example, don't practice on hard, wet, or uneven surfaces, and don't create pyramids that are more than two people high. And learn what to do in case of an injury or emergency.

- **Talk to your coach about any safety concerns,** or ask your parent or guardian to talk to your coach.

- **Learn how to help your teammates stay safe.** For sports like cheerleading or gymnastics, for example, learn how to be a good spotter.

- **Make sure to read about concussions.** Anyone who might have a head injury should not practice or compete until a health professional says it's safe.

- **Give your body a break.** Experts suggest the following:

- Take at least one day off per week from your sport or training schedule.

- Take at least two to three months off from your sport each year.

- If you train a lot in a high-impact sport, such as running, try replacing some intense training with lower-impact activities, such as biking.

- **Try different sports.** Playing the same sport over and over can put repeated stress on certain parts of your body. Doing a mix of sports and activities can help prevent this problem.

- **Strengthen your muscles.** Conditioning exercises, such as sit-ups and push-ups, can strengthen the muscles you use when you compete. Learn more about strengthening exercises.

- **Skip special supplements.** Products may claim to help you lose weight, bulk up, or improve your performance. Often these don't work, and they can even hurt you. Remember, all you really need to succeed is good nutrition.

Muscle Mistakes

Teen athletes sometimes try taking steroids to build their muscles and improve their performance. Using steroids in this way is illegal and dangerous. Steroids can cause problems with your periods and your heart, make hair grow on your face, and even change your behavior. That's not a very winning approach!

Chapter 27

Activities For Teens Who Don't Like Sports

Physical Activity And Teens[1]

According to the National Association for Sports and Physical Education (NASPE), children and teens should participate in a minimum of 60 minutes per day of daily moderate-to-vigorous physical activity, such as walking, running or playing basketball. Some children may not enjoy all the rules and competitive emphasis of organized sports. Rules can be confusing and often create a game that ends with winners and losers. Many activities involve group participation but not tough competition or awkward uniforms. Examples include tutoring, art and photography class, drama, school government, and walking in a charity walk-a-thon. However, sports like cheerleading or hockey offer great physical and social outlets for children inclined to team activities.

Guidelines For Children And Youth

The guidelines advise that:

- Children and youth do 60 minutes or more of physical activity every day. Activities should vary and be a good fit for their age and physical development. Children are naturally active, especially when they're involved in unstructured play (like recess). Any type of activity counts toward the advised 60 minutes or more.

About This Chapter: This chapter includes text excerpted from documents published by three public domain sources. Text under the headings marked 1 are excerpted from "Keep Active Without Keeping Score," Centers for Disease Control and Prevention (CDC), June 20, 2017; Text under the heading marked 2 is excerpted from "Being A Team Player Can Influence Drug And Alcohol Use," National Institute on Drug Abuse (NIDA), June 20, 2012. Reviewed September 2017; Text under the heading marked 3 is excerpted from "10 Tips: Stay Fit On Campus," ChooseMyPlate.gov, U.S. Department of Agriculture (USDA), February 16, 2017.

- Most physical activity should be moderate-intensity aerobic activity. Examples include walking, running, skipping, playing on the playground, playing basketball, and biking.
- Vigorous-intensity aerobic activity should be included at least 3 days a week. Examples include running, doing jumping jacks, and fast swimming.
- Muscle-strengthening activities should be included at least 3 days a week. Examples include playing on playground equipment, playing tug-of-war, and doing pushups and pullups.
- Bone-strengthening activities should be included at least 3 days a week. Examples include hopping, skipping, doing jumping jacks, playing volleyball, and working with resistance bands.

Children and youth who have disabilities should work with their doctors to find out what types and amounts of physical activity are safe for them. When possible, these children should meet the recommendations in the guidelines.

Some experts also advise that children and youth reduce screen time because it limits time for physical activity. They recommend that children aged 2 and older should spend no more than 2 hours a day watching television or using a computer (except for school work).

(Sources: "Recommendations For Physical Activity," National Heart, Lung, and Blood Institute (NHLBI).)

Knowing The Facts Leads To Winning Choices[2]

Middle and high school teens have many choices when it comes to extracurricular activities. Some will choose a team sport like basketball, volleyball, football, or softball, while others may choose more individual-type sports like track, golf, tennis, or swimming. Either way, being an athlete can be a positive experience—it teaches the importance of cooperation and practice, and how to win and lose gracefully—and it helps keep your body healthy. A recent study reports it may also influence decisions about using drugs like cigarettes, marijuana, or alcohol—but the news is not all good.

The good news is that researchers found that students who participate in team sports or exercise regularly report much less cigarette smoking than students not involved in sports. Also, fewer student athletes used marijuana.

The bad news is that the same study showed the reverse when it comes to drinking alcohol—that student athletes were much more likely to drink alcohol than nonathletes. This may be because team sports often involve alcohol—while watching the event or celebrating afterwards. That's why beer companies are major sponsors of pro sports teams.

Whether you play sports or not, making healthy choices is up to you. So, think about this: Are you more likely to drink or smoke if your friends do? How does being part of a team or group influence you?

How Can You Beat Boredom And See A New Side To Staying Active?[1]

The U.S. Department of Health and Human Services' Centers for Disease Control and Prevention developed the following list of alternative activities you might enjoy.

Table 27.1. Alternative Activities

If You Like ...	Why Not Try ...
PUTTING Your Best Foot Forward	Karate, Tae Bo, Capoeira
WHEELING Around Town	Roller Skating, Roller Blading, Skateboarding
MARCHING to the Beat of a Different Drum	Playing in an Orchestra, Playing Guitar with Friends
ACTING Like an Animal	Rodeo, Equestrian, Leap Frog
STANDING Out in the Crowd	Drama, Group Tutoring, Vocational Clubs
CREATING Your Own Masterpiece	Photography Club, Sculpting, Painting, Building a Fort
EXPERIMENTING with Nature	Measuring Your Heart Rate after Running Planting a Garden with Your Parents Rock Collecting at the Local Park
LIVING on the Edge	Riding a Dirt Bike, Skiing, Snowboarding
TAKING It Easy	Fishing, Yoga, Ballet
TESTING Your Limits	Archery, Hiking, Surfing
PLAYING Around the Neighborhood	Hacky Sack, Kick Ball, Tetherba

Ten Tips: Stay Fit On Campus[3]

Between classes and studying, it can be difficult to find time to be active. Even if you only exercise for a short period of time, you will feel more energized and better about your health. Get up and move!

1. **Walk or bike to class**

   If you live close enough to campus, avoid driving or spending money on public transportation by walking or biking to class. If you drive to campus, park your car farther away from the building to lengthen your walk.

2. **Take the stairs**

   As tempting as the elevators and escalators are, avoid them by using the stairs. This exercise is a great habit to start and will help tone your legs at the same time!

3. **Join a sport**

   Find a sport that interests you the most and one that will keep you active during your spare time. If you played a sport in high school such as basketball or soccer, you can continue playing in college!

4. **Join an intramural team**

   Another fun way to remain active is by joining an intramural team. Most universities offer classic sports such as basketball or baseball. But some campuses also offer activities such as ultimate frisbee and bowling.

5. **Hit the gym!**

   Visit your school's gym or recreation center. Go for a run on an indoor track or grab a basketball and shoot some hoops. Try to vary your routine each time to avoid boredom.

6. **Be active with friends**

   Go for a walk, hike, or bike ride with friends to catch up and have fun!

7. **Take a fitness class**

   Most universities offer a wide range of fitness classes for little or no charge. Find a schedule online and choose a class that you enjoy such as yoga, spinning, kickboxing, or aerobics.

8. **Fitness for credit**

   Elective classes such as swimming are a great way to remain active while also earning school credit. Not only are these classes fun, but they offer you a scheduled workout once or twice a week. Sign up with friends or try out a new class that strikes your interest.

9. **Sign up for an adventure trip**

   Many universities also offer adventure trips, such as hiking and whitewater rafting, to their students at a discounted price.

10. **Balance calories!**

    What you eat is just as important as how active you are. Keep track of how much you eat and your daily physical activity to help you to maintain a healthy weight.

Chapter 28

Baseball And Softball

Baseball

Just what does it take to become a baseball All-star?

Gear Up

All ball players will need a ball, a bat, and a glove. All baseballs are pretty much the same, but bats can be either wooden or aluminum. These days, only the pros use wooden bats full time. Aluminum bats are lighter and easier to handle and don't break as often. There are a couple of different types of gloves, depending on your field position.

Batter up! All batters should wear a helmet while at the plate and on base to protect the head. For better base running, try wearing baseball cleats instead of sneakers.

What a catch! Catchers have a special set of protective gear that includes a helmet, a mask, shin guards, and a chest protector. All of these pieces are very important to protect you if you play behind the plate.

Play It Safe

Wear your protective gear during all practices and games, especially if you're a catcher—those fast balls can pack a punch! Don't forget to warm up and stretch before each practice or game. In the infield? Stay behind the base on any throw. You'll avoid hurting yourself—and the base runner. In the outfield? Avoid bloopers with your teammates by calling every fly ball

About This Chapter: Text under the heading "Baseball" is excerpted from "BAM! Body And Mind—Baseball Activity Card," Centers for Disease Control and Prevention (CDC), May 9, 2015; Text under the heading "Softball" is excerpted from "BAM! Body And Mind—Softball Activity Card," Centers for Disease Control and Prevention (CDC), May 9, 2015.

loudly, even if you think nobody else is close by. And in the batter's' box, wear a batting helmet and use a batting glove to protect your knuckles from those inside pitches. If you think a pitch is going to hit you, turn away from the ball and take it in the back.

Throwing those fastballs can really take a toll, so if you're a pitcher, make sure to get plenty of rest between games, and don't pitch more than 4–10 innings per week.

How To Play

Baseball is known as America's favorite pastime. This sport uses many different skills from pitching, catching, and batting (which require lots of hand-eye coordination), to base running which means going from a standing start to a full sprint. To get started, you just need a bat and a ball!

How To Hit The Ball

First, get hold of that bat by stacking your hands on the handle (right hand on top if you're a righty, left hand on top if you're a lefty), making sure the curve of the bat is in the middle of your fingers and that your knuckles are in a straight line. Balance on the balls of your feet, with your weight on your back foot, and bend your knees slightly. Your hands should be shoulder height, elbows in, and keep your head in line with your torso, turned toward your front shoulder. As the pitcher throws, step toward the pitch, and swivel toward the ball with your hips, keeping your arms steady as you move toward the ball. Keep Your Eye On The Ball, and complete your swing by pivoting forward and shifting your weight to your front foot, following through with the bat after you hit the ball.

How To Throw The Ball

Did you know that throwing the ball accurately requires a little footwork? First, step toward the target with the glove side foot, making sure the toe of your shoe is pointing directly to where you want the ball to go. Aim the leading shoulder at the target. Aim the bill of your hat (the "duckbill") at the target and throw.

How To Catch The Ball

Keep your eye on the pitch and stay low with your feet apart and knees bent so you can move quickly in any direction. Have your glove ready at or below knee level, pocket side out. When scooping up a ground ball, bend down and use both hands to scoop it to the middle of your body so you have it securely.

Ology

How does Barry Bonds hit the ball so far? It's science! When the bat hits the ball, the bat exchanges momentum with the ball and the ball takes off. The faster the bat is swung, the harder it hits the ball and the harder the bat hits the ball, the faster and further the ball goes. So if you want to hit like Barry, pump up those arm muscles and take some practice swings!

Softball

Do you want to be a softball all-star?

Gear Up

You'll need a glove that fits your hand and skill level, and is geared to the position you play. There's a lot of truth to the old saying, "Fits like a glove"—if you're glove is too big, or small, you may have problems catching and fielding the ball. For beginners, gloves that are about 9 1/2 to 11 inches long are a good start.

You can't play without a bat and ball! Try aluminum or other non-wooden bats—they are lighter and easier to handle. As for the ball, you can find softballs at most stores that sell sports equipment.

Also, for organized team play, you'll need a pair of shoes with rubber cleats—they dig into the ground and can give you more traction while running the bases or fielding a ball. If you're playing a pickup game with your friends, a pair of sneakers will do. If you're a catcher, you'll need special protective gear like a helmet with a facemask, shin guards, and a chest protector.

And remember, always wear a helmet to protect your head while at the plate, or on base!

Play It Safe

Before you hit the field, Warm Up! Get all of your muscles ready to play by stretching before every game.

Whether you're in the field or up to bat, don't forget to wear your safety gear in games and in practices. A helmet is important when batting, waiting to bat, or running the bases. If you're a catcher, make sure you wear your protective gear during all practices and games, and wear it properly—have your coach or a parent check it out for you. Don't wear jewelry like rings, watches, or necklaces—they could cut you (or someone else), or get caught when you're running the bases.

Did you know that an umpire could call you out for throwing your bat? Well, they can! And, it's not just the out you have to worry about—it's your teammates' safety! Always drop your bat next to your side in the batter's box before you head for first base.

Be a team player—always know where your teammates are before throwing the ball or swinging your bat. Make sure they are ready and have their glove up as a target before you throw the ball to them. Call loudly for every fly ball or pop up in the field, even if you don't think any of your teammates are close by. Teams that play together win together!

How To Play

Softball is a game of speed, skill, and smarts! Whether you're looking to play in your backyard or at the state championships, softball is a great team sport that everyone can play!

Many of the skills in softball are similar to those in baseball, but there are some unique differences that make softball a game of its own!

Did you know that a softball isn't really soft at all, and that it's almost two times bigger than a baseball? Because a softball is kinda' big, it doesn't go as far when you hit it. But, keep your eye on the ball—a softball can sometimes cross the plate at a very fast speed! Even with their underhanded pitching style (unlike baseball's overhand style), softball pitchers can put a lot of heat on the ball. Most beginners play in slow pitch leagues where the hitting game is having a sharp eye and timing your swing. Keep your eyes peeled for pitches that are shoulder high and that drop right over the plate—they are perfect for driving into the field.

If you're interested in playing at a more competitive level, fast-pitch softball is what you'll see—you can steal bases and bunt, and you only need nine players to get a game going. If you're playing a pickup game with your friends, you'll probably play slow pitch softball. You only need ten players to field a team, but invite as many people as you want—it's more fun that way!

Ology

Did you know that it's easier to hit a home run in outer space? That's because the density (thickness) of the air on earth plays a role in how far a ball travels when it's been hit. The particles that make up air on earth are close together—this makes it difficult for things (like a softball) to travel through it. If you took away the air altogether, the ball would keep going. In places like Colorado where the altitude (height of the land above water level) is higher, the air is thinner, and a ball can fly much farther. Under these conditions, a hit that might be a routine fly ball can sail over the fence with no problem.

Chapter 29

Basketball

Just what does it take to become a basketball star?

Gear Up

A Basketball. Basketballs come in different sizes depending on your age and whether you're a girl or boy. There are also different basketballs for inside and outside use. If you're buying a new basketball, make sure you ask the salesperson for help to figure out what size and type ball you need.

A Hoop. Basketball hoops are available in most gyms and in many parks. You can even buy a hoop and attach it to the side of your house or garage, if you have one. To create your own regulation court at your house, make sure you set your foul line 15 feet from the backboard.

Play It Safe

Basketball can really make you work, so make sure you stretch and warm up before playing. Because of all of the quick moves and jumping, it can put a lot of wear and tear on your ankles, so protect them by wearing the right pair of shoes—medium or high tops do the best job of supporting your ankles. Protect those knees by learning how to cut, stop, and land a jump safely.

Be careful not to misuse basketball equipment. It's great if you've got the skills to put up a mean slam dunk, but hanging on the rim is dangerous and could cause you to get hurt. Also, make sure the court and sidelines are clear of any obstacles such as other basketballs or water bottles. If you're playing outside, make sure the baskets and sidelines are not too close to walls, fences, or bleachers and there are no holes on your court.

About This Chapter: This chapter includes text excerpted from "BAM! Body And Mind—Basketball Activity Card," Centers for Disease Control and Prevention (CDC), May 9, 2015.

If you're a serious player, you may want to invest in a mouth guard to keep your teeth safe from flying elbows; knee and elbow pads so you don't get scraped up (especially if you're playing on an outdoor court); and sports glasses to protect your eyes.

> Concussion is a possible risk for those who play basketball, soccer, lacrosse, and other sports. To lower the chances of getting a concussion, always make sure to follow any rules of your sport and to use the right equipment.
>
> *(Source: "Physical Activity Safety Tips For Girls—Avoiding Injuries," girlshealth.gov, Office on Women's Health (OWH).)*

How To Play

Basketball is fun to play in pickup games in the yard with your pals, or you can join an organized league. Different positions rely on different skills—point guards should focus on their dribbling and passing, while centers and forwards should be powerful rebounders and shooters. Outside guards need to be quick and strong to make those 3-point shots. Want some basics?

- **How to dribble.** Bounce the ball on the floor with your strongest arm. When it bounces back, use your fingertips to stop the upward motion and push it back to the floor, keeping it about waist high when it bounces. Once you've mastered dribbling in place with one hand, switch to the other and begin to move around as you dribble. Practicing dribbling by moving the ball in a figure eight between your legs is one good way to build your skills.

- **How to pass the ball.** Face the person you're passing to, with your head up and knees slightly bent. Spread your fingers wide and hold the ball at chest level, elbows out. Extend your arms, take a step toward the person you're passing to, and snap your wrists forward and up as you release the ball.

- **How to shoot a layup.** Start about 10 feet in front of and to the right of the basket. Dribble toward the basket, timing it so that your last step is with your left foot. Holding the ball with both hands (left in front, right in back), jump off your left foot, let go with your left hand, and extend your right arm fully to release the ball at the top of your jump. Keeping your eyes on where you want the ball to go really helps land this shot!

- **How to cut, stop, and land a jump.** Ease up on your cuts or pivots by making them less sharp to avoid rotating your knees. When stopping, rather than coming to a sudden stop or bringing your weight down on one foot with a single step, use the "stutter step" to slow yourself down by taking two extra steps. When landing your jumps, do it softly by bending your knees over your feet (which should be pointed straight ahead) when you hit the ground. Instead of landing flat-footed, land on either the balls or toes of your feet and rock back toward your heels.

Ology

Did you ever wonder how Michael Jordan seems to hang in the air longer than everyone else when he goes up for a slam dunk? Well, actually, he doesn't—it just seems that way because MJ holds onto the ball longer than most players before shooting or dunking. Hang time depends entirely on the force generated by a player's legs when he or she leaves the ground (how hard they push off the ground) and the jump's height (the higher the jump, the longer the hang time). The average National Basketball Association (NBA) player can make a 3-foot high jump when going up for a shot or dunk, with a hang time of less than 1 second (.87 seconds to be exact).

Chapter 30

Bicycling And Indoor Cycling

Just what does it take to become a cyclist?

Gear Up

A Bike. Think of the type of riding you want to do before you buy one. Mountain bikes are strong and stable and built for gravel roads and tricky trails. Racing bikes are built to go super-fast on pavement, and sport bikes, a combination of both, are good for many different purposes.

A Helmet. Your helmet should sit right above your eyebrows and be tightly buckled so it doesn't slip while you are riding.

Play It Safe

Use your head and wear a helmet! You should always wear a helmet when you ride—plus, it's the law in many states. It's also important that your helmet is approved by one of the groups who test helmets to see which ones are the best: the Consumer Product Safety Commission (CPSC) or Snell B-95 standards are best for bicycling helmets. Try not to ride at night or in bad weather, and wear brightly colored, or reflective clothes whenever you ride so you can be seen. You can even put reflectors or funky reflective stickers on your bike—who knew being safe could look so cool? Also, watch out for loose pant legs and shoe laces that could get caught in your bike chain.

About This Chapter: This chapter includes text excerpted from "BAM! Body And Mind—Bicycling Activity Card," Centers for Disease Control and Prevention (CDC), May 9, 2015.

Be street smart. Ride on the right side of the road, moving with traffic, and obey all traffic signs and signals. Discuss the best riding routes with your parents—they'll help you determine safe places to ride near your home.

When you reach an intersection, be sure to stop and look left, right, and then left again to check for cars—then go. Use hand signals to show when you're going to turn, and be sure to keep an eye out for rough pavement ahead so you can avoid it. And although you may think you can't go out without your favorite tunes, never wear headphones when you're on your bike.

How To Play

Bicycling can be a great competitive sport, as well as a fun activity to do with your friends. And there are plenty of different types of bicycling depending on your personality. If you love to go fast-n-furious, bicycle racing is probably more your speed. If you like to hit the rocky road, mountain biking sounds more like your taste. And if you just like to pedal for pleasure, any kind of bicycling will do. Try riding to school or to a friend's house!

Ology

The faster you are going, the longer it will take you to completely stop your bike once you hit the brakes. Science says that if you are going 20 miles per hour and you hit the brakes, it will take 15 feet to stop if you are on dry pavement, and 23 1/2 feet if you are on wet pavement, so make sure you brake early!

Chapter 31

Football

Just what does it take to become a football All-star?

Gear Up

Obviously, you need a football to play, and you should choose the size based on your age. Always wear a helmet with a face mask and jaw pads, and a mouthpiece to protect against those hard hits. Because football is a contact sport, there are many different pieces of gear you should wear to protect different areas of your body. For upper body protection, you should wear a neck roll to prevent whiplash, shoulder pads, rib pads, arm pads, and elbow pads. For leg protection, you should wear hip pads, tailbone pads, thigh pads, and knee pads. Most leagues require all this, but it's a good idea to protect yourself even in backyard games.

Play It Safe

Be sure to stretch and warm up before every practice and game and always wear your protective gear. To avoid getting hurt, learn from your coaches how to block and tackle correctly. Don't tackle with the top of your head or helmet—not only is it illegal, but it can cause injury to both players. If you play in an organized league, there are lots of rules—and they are there for a reason—to keep you safe. If you break these rules, you risk not only getting hurt, or hurting someone else, but your team will be penalized. If you're playing in the backyard with your friends, stay safe by sticking to touch or flag football, and only play with kids who are around your age and size.

About This Chapter: This chapter includes text excerpted from "BAM! Body And Mind—Football Activity Card," Centers for Disease Control and Prevention (CDC), May 9, 2015.

How To Play

There are lots of skills needed to play football from throwing and catching the ball to blocking and tackling the other players. There's even a national Punt, Pass, and Kick contest devoted just to the main skills you need. League teams are a great way to learn all the rules and strategies of football. Pop Warner is the most popular youth football league, but there are many others nationwide. Want the basics?

- **Throwing the ball.** Grip the ball by placing each of your fingers between each lace of the ball. Bring your throwing arm back with your elbow bent. Extend your free arm (the one without the ball) in front of you and point to your target. Snap your throwing arm forward, releasing the ball, and follow through with your shoulders and hips. When you are finished, your throwing arm should be pointing toward your target with your palm facing the ground.

- **Catching the ball.** Hold your arms out with your elbows slightly bent in front of your chest. Bring your hands together, touching the thumbs and index fingers to make a triangle with your fingers. Catch the nose of the ball in the triangle, and use your chest to help trap the ball. Bring your arms in around the ball and hold it tight against you.

- **Punting the ball.** Place your feet shoulder-width apart with your kicking foot slightly in front. Slightly bend your knees and bend your body forward a little. Hold the ball out in front of you with the laces facing upward. Take two steps forward, beginning with your kicking foot and drop the ball toward your kicking foot. Kick the ball hard with the top of your foot and follow through with your leg as high as you can.

Ology

You'd think more football players would study physics, since how far you can throw a football is definitely a science. How far a football goes is a combination of the "velocity" or speed of the football after you throw it, the angle (or arc) the football is thrown at, and how the ball rotates in the air (that's why it's best to throw a spiral).

Chapter 32

Frisbee

Just what does it take to play frisbee?

Gear Up

Of course the first thing you'll need is a frisbee! The most common kinds are made of plastic and come in all sorts of cool colors. If you are planning to play a serious game, or want to play an organized game of Ultimate, you'll also need cleats or tennis shoes with good tread. Kneepads aren't a bad idea and are a great way to avoid scratching up your knees.

Play It Safe

When playing a game of frisbee, just make sure that you don't throw too hard and always try and stay on your feet while playing. If you are playing a more intense game of Ultimate also make sure to avoid diving for the frisbee.

It's important to warm up and stretch before any game. Listen to your body! Don't play through any pain. If you are injured, wait until you've healed before starting to play again. And if you have glasses or braces, wear protective eye or mouth guards.

Whether you're just tossing the frisbee with friends or playing a competitive game of Ultimate, make sure to drink plenty of water before, during and after your game. It's also a good idea to wear sunscreen to keep from burning and bug repellent to keep the bugs where they belong—off of you!

About This Chapter: This chapter includes text excerpted from "BAM! Body And Mind—Frisbee Activity Card," Centers for Disease Control and Prevention (CDC), May 9, 2015.

How To Play

Frisbee is a great way to spend time outside on a beautiful day. Just grab your frisbee and a few friends and you've got yourself a game!

One of the best parts about frisbee is that you probably know more than you think about how to play! Like how to throw a backhand: Just stand with your feet shoulder-width apart, point yourself sideways, place your index finger on the outside rim with your middle finger extended along the top of the frisbee and your thumb underneath and flick your wrist toward your throwing partner.

A forehanded frisbee throw is more complicated, but just remember—practice makes perfect! Place your middle finger straight and flat against the inside rim of the frisbee so that the outer rim is between your thumb and your index finger. If you are right handed, stand sideways with your left shoulder forward, pull your right arm back to your outer thigh, keeping the frisbee at an angle, and flick your wrist forward, releasing the frisbee about halfway across your body.

Now that you've perfected throwing the frisbee, you've got to learn to catch it. There are two ways to catch a frisbee. In one, called the "Pancake," the palms of your hands face each other and are held close to your body. That way, if you can't catch the frisbee with your hands, it hits your body, not the ground. Another catch style is called the "Crocodile." This catch involves holding your arms out in front of your body and clapping your hands together just like a crocodile's mouth snapping shut.

Once you've mastered catching and throwing your frisbee, grab some friends and organize a game of Ultimate! This is a team sport played on a 70-yard by 40-yard rectangular field with an end zone that stretches 25 yards deep. Two teams of seven people each are needed to play. A team scores when the frisbee is thrown into the other team's end zone. Ultimate players referee their own games, making good sportsmanship the most important thing to remember!

Ology

If you want to make your frisbee soar, make sure you put lots of spin on it when you throw. Spinning helps keep the frisbee from flipping over, which would put an end to your throw. Frisbee designers help you by making the edges thicker than the rest of the frisbee and by putting tiny ridges on the top to help keep it balanced.

Chapter 33

Golf

Just what does it take to play golf?

Gear Up

Don't worry about buying an entire set of golf clubs right away. If you're just starting out, all you really need are the 5, 6, or 7 irons, a driver, and a putter. You'll use a driver off of the tee for long distance shots, followed up by your irons, which give more control for shorter shots. And don't forget your putter—the putter is used on the green.

Next on your list should be golf balls and tees. Tees look like a round peg with a flat top, and are used to raise the ball off of the ground so you can get your club under it better. Put the tee into the ground and sit your golf ball on top of it. Make sure you have plenty of tees on hand—they sometimes break when you hit the ball. Don't get overwhelmed by the number of golf balls there are to choose from! You don't have to use an expensive ball because a lot of them will probably end up in the woods or water anyway.

Also, don't forget that some courses have a dress code. This means that they can ask you to wear certain types of clothing like shirts with collars and shorts or pants without holes in them! As a rule of thumb, keep your clothing simple. Dress in comfortable, loose fitting shirts, pants, or shorts. Sneakers are fine for beginners. And don't forget a hat and sunscreen! On those hot, sunny days, it's important to protect yourself from the sun.

Once you've got all of your gear, hit the links and have some fun!

About This Chapter: This chapter includes text excerpted from "BAM! Body And Mind—Golf Activity Card," Centers for Disease Control and Prevention (CDC), May 9, 2015.

Play It Safe

It's important to warm-up and stretch before you step onto your local golf course. Before swinging, make sure that no one is standing too close—it's a good rule of thumb to stand at least four club lengths away from the person swinging the club. Don't play until the group in front of you is out of the way. Stand still and stay quiet while others are in play. If your ball lands in the rough of the course (in high grass, brush, or trees), watch out for creepy, crawly animals and poisonous plants.

Check the weather forecast before going out onto the course. The general rule for avoiding storms is: If you can see lightning, flee it, if you can hear thunder, clear it. Get away from small metal vehicles like golf carts, and put your clubs away. Stay away from trees because they attract lightning, and avoid small on-course shelters—they are made to protect you from rain showers and provide shade.

Whether you're walking the course or riding in a cart, don't forget your water bottle. It's important to drink plenty of water before, during, and after your round. Need a rest? Sit down in a shady area, or under a tree—put a cold towel around your neck to keep you cool.

How To Play

Golf is played on a course with either nine or 18 different holes—a complete game of golf is called a round. It's important to know the basics of the game and how to use (and choose) your clubs. You may want to take a few lessons from the pro at your local golf course, or rent an instructional video to learn more about the proper swing, grip, and stance.

Check out these tips to get you swingin' in the right direction.

- **The clubs.** If your clubs are too long or too short, you're likely to have problems. To find the right size clubs for you, try swinging with a few different lengths. A good rule of thumb is to choose clubs that are about as long as the distance from your bellybutton to the floor. You don't need to decide right away—lots of courses and driving ranges have sample clubs that you can practice with until you find the perfect fit!

- **The swing.** The key to the swing is to keep your eyes on the ball. Focus on the ball and keep your head down (and still) when you swing. Your eyes should stay on the ball through your entire swing.

Jack Nicklaus, one of the best players in golf, learned one basic thing from his father—hit the ball hard, and not worry about where it goes—you can always fix that later. By trying to hit the ball far, you'll naturally try to make the biggest swing with your arms that you can. Swing them back as far as you can—getting your hands behind your head, and follow through as far as you can. You'll feel your body turn and you'll notice that while swinging back, your weight will shift to your right foot, and then to your left as you swing through the ball.

- **Tee it up.** If you're a beginner, hit the ball off of a tee every time—it's much easier to get under the ball. Put the tee into the ground at different heights to see where you like it best. If you're a more experienced player, only use a tee when using your drivers. Experiment with your irons once you're in the fairway to get the ball onto the green. Just remember that the iron you choose depends on how far (and high) you need to hit the ball. Use a 3 iron for long shots to the hole—a 9 iron can be used for those shorter shots.

Ology

Did you know that the dimples on a golf ball make it travel farther? It has to do with air flow. As air flows around a ball without dimples, it breaks away from the surface of the ball forming a pocket of swirling currents behind it—like the wake behind a speedboat. This creates a "drag" on the ball, slowing it down. Dimpled golf balls can easily sail two hundred yards from the tee, while a smooth one (with no dimples) would only go about fifty yards! Golfers discovered this about a hundred years ago, when they noticed their old golf balls, covered with scratches and nicks, sailed farther down the fairway than shiny new ones.

Chapter 34

Gymnastics, Cheerleading, And Ballet

Gymnastics

Just what does it take to do gymnastics?

Gear Up

Unlike some other sports, gymnastics doesn't require a lot of equipment, but there are certain things you'll need for specific events, and some standard gear that all gymnasts should have.

Female gymnasts usually wear leotards (one or two piece outfits that fit snuggly to the body). Boys can wear running shorts or sweatpants with fitted tops, or with your shirt tucked in. Just make sure you don't wear clothing that is too loose—it could get caught on the equipment when you are performing your tricks and cause you serious problems! For those of you with long locks, you'll need to pull it back with a hair band or in a braid—this will prevent it from getting in your face during your routine which could cause you to lose concentration and sight.

Gymnasts also wear hand guards and use chalk to prevent their hands from slipping when working on the floor mats, rings, or bars. The hand guards help prevent blisters and make it easier to swing around on the bars.

About This Chapter: Text under the heading "Gymnastics" is excerpted from "BAM! Body And Mind—Gymnastics Activity Card," Centers for Disease Control and Prevention (CDC), May 9, 2015; Text under the heading "Cheerleading" is excerpted from "BAM! Body And Mind—Cheerleading Activity Card," Centers for Disease Control and Prevention (CDC), May 9, 2015; Text under the heading "Ballet" is excerpted from "BAM! Body And Mind—Ballet Activity Card," Centers for Disease Control and Prevention (CDC), May 9, 2015.

Play It Safe

The most important gymnastics rule to remember is to know what you're doing! Never attempt a trick you are not familiar with. Make sure you always have a trained spotter (someone who stands near you in case you need help while doing your tricks) just in case you lose your balance on the beam, or attempt a wobbly handstand.

Before you attempt any trick or stunt, always make sure the equipment is sturdy and has been set up properly (always ask a coach or another grownup for help). Floors should be padded with mats that are secured under every piece of equipment. Also, make sure there is enough distance between each piece of equipment before you start swingin'! Collisions can cause you, or others around you, to get hurt if you don't watch out. Use your head! Pay attention and be serious about your practice—horseplay and goofing around can get you into trouble! Always know what your teammates are doing and where they are.

And last but not least, never eat or chew gum while doing gymnastics—the moment you become unaware of what is in your mouth, it can easily become lodged in your throat and you could choke!

How To Play

Gymnastics is known as the sport of all sports. It's a great way to improve strength, flexibility, balance, and coordination for other types of physical activities, and it's a great way to meet new people and have fun!

It doesn't matter if you're a guy or a girl—gymnastics has a few different categories to choose from so you can find your favorite. Artistic gymnasts use lots of skills to perform on many different kinds of apparatuses (pieces of equipment). Boys participate in six events (floor, vault, parallel bars, high bar, still rings, and pommel horse) and girls in four (floor, vault, uneven parallel bars, and balance beam). Gymnasts who participate in rhythmic gymnastics jump, tumble, flip, and dance to music while using rope, hoops, bars, or ribbons as part of their routines. In gymnastics, there's something for everyone!

But, before you get started, you need to know (and master) the basics!

The handstand is one of the basic skills of gymnastics. If you're a beginner, it's a good idea to practice your handstands against a wall until you get your balance and build up your strength and confidence. And remember, it is always good to have a spotter—just in case you need some help along the way!

Follow these tips to a perfect handstand:

- Face the wall.

- Get in a squatted position so that your knees are bent and your body is close to the ground.

- Put your hands on the floor with the tips of your fingers facing the wall (your hands should not be any wider than shoulder width apart).

- Bend your head down to the floor—keeping it between your arms.

- Kick your legs up putting all your weight on your hands—keeping your upper body straight and tight.

- Once your feet hit the wall, straighten out your legs.

Now that you've mastered the handstand—wanna' try something trickier?

Practice these steps to conquer the cartwheel:

- Stand in a ready position, your "favorite" leg in front, knees bent slightly. To find out your favorite leg, stand up and take one step. The leg you step forward with first is usually your favorite.

- Raise both of your arms.

- Reach forward with your right arm, putting your right hand on the floor/ground.

- Shift your weight to your right arm and kick your left leg up (If you're a lefty, reverse these directions).

- Your left hand should follow very quickly—as it touches the ground, shift your weight to your left arm. Your right leg should be off of the ground.

- Bring your left leg down, right hand up, right leg down, left hand up.

Ology

Did you know that you could lose weight by doing handstands? You can—but it's only temporary. Many athletes who have to "weigh in" before competitions such as wrestlers, weight lifters, or rowers do handstands for about two minutes against a wall before they step on the scale. While they're upside down, all of the blood rushes to their head. When they step on the scale, the blood is in free fall, causing it to be weightless and the athlete a few pounds lighter!

Cheerleading

Just what does it take to do cheerleading?

Gear Up

You'll need a good comfortable pair of sneakers that provide a lot of support and cushion for your feet. Also, many cheerleaders use spirit-raising tools such as pom-pons and megaphones.

Play It Safe

Today's cheerleading is super fun, but it's risky too—especially if you perform stunts. On this team sport, each squad member's position is key to completing the stunts safely and dazzling the crowd.

Make sure you're well conditioned for all those kicks, jumps, and splits. Warm up before each practice and game, and do lots of stretching. Focus on stretching your legs and back. If you do stunts and build pyramids, make sure you stretch your arms and shoulders too!

Practice safe stunts! If your squad does lifts, tosses, or builds pyramids, make sure you follow these important safety rules.

Stunt Safety

- Always practice stunts on mats or pads.
- Never attempt a stunt unless a coach is there.
- Always use spotters for each and every stunt.
- If you are new to stunting, start with easier stunts and gradually move up to harder ones.
- Remember that if someone in the stunt yells "Down," the stunt should come down immediately.

How To Play

When you hear the word "cheerleading," what do you think of? How about a fast-paced competitive sport for both guys and girls that involves a high level of endurance, strength and precision? For many cheerleaders, that is exactly what cheering is. Cheerleading is coming into its own as a competitive sport. Cheer squads compete up to the national level, developing cheer and dance routines that include complex pyramids, lifts and tosses.

If you're just starting out, here are some basic cheerleading motions:

Arm Motions

- Goal Post. Arms should be above your head, straight up in the air, and touching the side of your head. Your fists should be closed with your thumbs facing each other.

- High V. From the goal post position, move your arms out slightly wider to form a high V. Fists should be closed and thumbs facing away from your body. Your arms should be slightly in front of you so that you can see your fists out of the corner of your eyes.

- Low V. For this motion, the opposite of a high V, move your arms down into a v-like position by your sides. Keep your fists closed with your thumbs facing away from your body.

- Basic T. Your arms should be straight out on each side, in line with your shoulders. Keep your fists closed with your thumbs facing down, and your arms straight and level. Your body should look like a T.

Jump Tips

There are four main parts to a jump:

- **The Prep.** Begin with your feet together with your weight on your toes. Move your arms to a high V position and keep your shoulders back.

- **The Whip.** Next, lift your body up through your shoulders, quickly swinging your arms forward in a circle. Bend at the knees, keeping on the balls of your feet, building up to the lift.

- **The Lift.** When your arms complete their circle to the high V position, jump off the ground, pushing through your toes. Once you are in the air, pull your legs up toward your arms. Keep your toes pointed, your arms stiff, and your head up.

- **The Landing.** Bring your legs together quickly so that your feet are together when they hit the ground. Bend your knees slightly to absorb the weight and take the pressure of your legs.

Ballet

Just what does it take to become a ballet All-star?

Gear Up

Tutus and toe shoes are a classical dancer's standard costume. When trying to figure out what to wear, keep in mind the following tips:

A simple leotard with tights is best for class—wearing them allows the instructor to see that all muscles are moving correctly. Boys often wear black tights and a white t-shirt.

In order to keep their muscles warm and help prevent injuries, sometimes dancers wear leg warmers for warming up and doing exercises at the barre. A barre is a handrail that dancers use to steady themselves during the first part of a ballet class. ("Barre" is also a shorthand term for exercises done at the barre, and you might hear a dancer say they are "doing a barre" before performing which means they are warming up).

Ordinary ballet shoes have paper-thin soles, no heels, are held on the foot with elastic and come in different colors (but usually black or pink). The right and left foot shoes are identical and take on the shape of each foot through use.

Pointe shoes have reinforced toes that help the toes bear the weight of the body and provide extra support for dancers going up on Pointe. Pointe places a lot of force on the toes, and the reinforcement also help distribute this pressure over the entire tip of the foot. But even then, dancers usually add padding inside the shoe to cushion their feet further. It's important that dancers don't wear toe or point shoes until their ankles, back and other supporting muscles are strong enough for this type of exercise—remember that Pointe is not for beginners! It's always best to go to a store that specializes in dancewear to have shoes fitted properly. A dancer's toes should be able to move freely inside while the shoe is snug and secure on the outside.

It's usually best to leave jewelry like watches, necklaces and dangling earrings at home. They could scratch another dancer or snag a leotard or tights, and might turn out to be a hassle.

Wearing your hair up for class allows your instructor to fully see how your muscles are aligned—and it helps you see where you are going!

Play It Safe

Stretching is one of the most important things a dancer can do. Stretching makes the muscles stronger and more flexible, so make sure you warm up and stay focused while stretching.

To prevent toe trouble, wear toe pads and tape around tender and tight parts of your feet like your toes and heels.

Learn the proper technique. To ensure correct technique, make sure you are being taught by a qualified teacher with proper credentials and that you practice under supervision.

Eat healthy in order to keep your energy and attention levels up so that you can perform at your best. Some dancers confuse healthy eating with not eating enough and develop eating disorders. It's never a good idea to try and make yourself skinny by hurting your body.

Ballet is more than just physical exertion. It's the total process of expressing yourself through creative movement—have confidence in your self expression and in everything else you do!

Simple crunches, lunges and bike riding are good ways to strengthen back muscles. You can also stretch your back muscles by lying on your stomach, slightly lifting both arms and legs and holding them in place for a few seconds.

How To Play

Confidence, good posture, balance, self-discipline, concentration, flexibility, endurance, speed, strength, and power. Would you believe there's a single activity that promotes all these things at the same time?! Well, believe it or not, there is—ballet!

There are two types of classic ballet, which is an art form that tells stories through characters in costume. Pointe is one type, where dancers wear a special type of shoe so that they can move on the tips of their toes. Since Pointe is really advanced, we'll just be focusing on demi-ballet. In this type, dancers dance on the balls of their feet.

There's a whole lot to remember when dancing ballet—things like how important it is to find the right studio. Because when you're learning the basics, it's important to make sure you learn correctly!

There are five basic positions for ballet. All classic dance steps start or end in one of these five positions:

- First Position—The heels are together, legs stretched straight. Turn your toes outward to form a straight line. You arms should form a curve raised right above your waist. Your hands should be between your waist and the level of your chest.

- Second Position—Separate your feet to the side about 1 ½ feet apart. Your feet should be well turned out. Open your arms, rounding them slightly. Your elbows should be slightly lower than your shoulders.

- Third Position—Put the heel of your right foot against the middle of your left foot. Bring your right arm up so that a semicircle forms above your head. Your left arm should remain in the second position.

- Fourth Position—Slide your right foot forward so that it is parallel to your left foot with about 12 inches in between. Place your right arm overhead in a vertical position. Your left arm should be in the first position.

- Fifth Position—Place your right foot close up in front of your left foot. The toes of your left foot should touch the heel of your right foot. Both arms should be overhead and form a round shape. There is a small space between hands.

In addition to the dancing done with their legs and feet, dancers use their hands and arms to express themselves. Showing expression through the hands and arms is always very important, especially since it can be difficult to see a dancer's face from a distance.

But the most important thing to remember—always respect the instructor!

Ology

Ancient man conveyed his thoughts, wishes, and emotions through actions, just as we do in modern ballets. In the Americas, Australia and Africa, aboriginal people danced both for spiritual reasons and for entertainment. Their dances continue to influence dance today.

Ballet was a man's game for many years, and men performed both male and female roles. Even when women were included, they weren't able to do some of the things men could, mainly because of their clothes. Men wore tights and were able to move freely, but women had to wear heavy wigs, huge headdresses, full skirts, high-heeled shoes and extra tight corsets that restricted breathing and bending. In addition to wearing uncomfortable clothing, women had to overcome society's disapproval of female performers as ballet moved from the ballroom to the stage.

Classical ballet came to America in the mid-1900s thanks to George Balanchine who founded the School of American Ballet in 1934, and later the New York City Ballet.

Chapter 35

Martial Arts

Who's that kid in the cool black belt?

Gear Up

Most martial arts students wear white pants, a white jacket, and a cloth belt. For some martial arts, the belt color shows the student's skill level and personal development—from white (beginner) to black (expert). The colors reflect nature. For example, the white belt that students start out with stands for a seed. The yellow belt that they get next stands for the sunshine that opens the seed. To advance from one grade level to another, you have to pass loads of tests—five for the green belt, nine for the brown belt, and 10 for the black belt! You can get a first-degree black belt in two to four years, but after that, there's still more to learn—There are 10 black belt levels!

For sparring (practice fighting), go for full gear, including a mouthpiece and padding on your head, hands, feet, and shins.

Play It Safe

Look for an instructor who's into respect and discipline, but still has plenty of patience. The class area should have lots of space and a smooth, flat floor with padding. The fewer students the better—more attention for you!

Wear all the right gear. Warm up and stretch so you're loose and ready to go! You need good instruction before launching into any moves. And when you do learn the moves, remember your limits. For example, white belt students shouldn't spar (practice fight).

About This Chapter: This chapter includes text excerpted from "BAM! Body And Mind—Martial Arts Activity Card," Centers for Disease Control and Prevention (CDC), May 9, 2015.

When you are ready for matches, you've gotta have an instructor around to regulate. Some martial artists use special weapons (like swords), but it's almost a sure thing that you'll get hurt with them unless you're totally advanced—so, no weapons. During your match, make sure that your partner knows when you're ready to stop. If you let your guard down, your partner may think it's a good chance to take you down!

How To Play

> Other martial arts include Aikido, Hwarang Do, Kung Fu, Jujitsu, Kendo, Ninjutsu, Northern and Southern Shaolin Boxing, Tai Chi, and T'an Su Do.
>
> **Interested?**
>
> The first thing you need to do is to decide on the style you want to study. Do you want to enter tournaments, or simply know how to defend yourself? After that, just get into a good class!

Martial arts—a special type of defense skills—started in the Orient (East Asia). Today, they're taught all over the world for self-defense and avoiding conflict, too. Body and mind control, discipline, and confidence are key. There are a lot of martial arts styles, but since certain types rough up the joints (like knees) more than others, these are some of the best for kids your age:

Judo comes from Japan and means "gentle way." It's like Jujitsu, one of the oldest martial arts, but not as hard core. Judo has lots of wrestling moves. It also teaches participants how to make good decisions and be mentally strong. Judokas (judo players) focus on competition.

Karate comes from Japan, and means "empty hand." It's Japan's most popular martial art. Feet, legs, elbows, head, and fists get used for kicking, punching, defensive blocks, and more. Karate stresses defense and uses weapons.

Tae Kwon Do comes from Korea and means "the way of the foot and fist." It's famous for high kicks. Tae Kwon Do became Korea's national sport in 1955 and is now the world's most popular martial art.

Ology

If you open your hands wide and shove something, your force spreads out across your palm and fingers. But if you hold all of your fingers together and hit with only the side of your hand or your fingertips, that same amount of force goes to a much smaller area and the hit is harder. If you try this on yourself, you'll see the difference. Just don't beat yourself up too much!

Chapter 36

Skating: Inline Skating And Skateboarding

Inline Skating

Just what does it take to do inline skating?

Gear Up

There are several different types of inline skates, depending on the type of skating you do. Recreational skates have a plastic boot and 4 wheels. These skates are best for beginners. Hockey skates have laces and are made of leather with small wheels for quick movement. Racing skates have 5 wheels and, usually, no brake. Freestyle skates have three wheels and a pick stop for tricks. Fitness skates have larger wheels and are used for cross-training. Aggressive skates, the kind worn by X Games competitors, are made of thick plastic with small wheels for quick movement, and grind plates to protect the skate when doing tricks. No matter what kind of skates you wear, always wear a helmet, as well as wrist guards, elbow pads, and knee pads

Play It Safe

Avoid getting hurt by making sure your helmet and pads are on correctly. Your helmet should be tightly buckled, with the front coming down to right over your eyebrow, and your pads should be on tight, so they don't slip while you are skating. It's also important that your helmet is approved by one of the groups who test helmets to see which ones are the best: the Consumer Product Safety Commission (CPSC), or Snell B-95 standards are best for inline

---

About This Chapter: Text under the heading "Inline Skating" is excerpted from "BAM! Body And Mind—Inline Skating Activity Card," Centers for Disease Control and Prevention (CDC), May 9, 2015; Text under the heading "Skateboarding" is excerpted from "BAM! Body And Mind—Skateboarding," Centers for Disease Control and Prevention (CDC), May 9, 2015.

skating helmets. Make sure you are always in control of your speed, turns and stops, and be careful of cracks in the pavement where you are skating—they can be dangerous if your wheels get caught in them. It's best to go skating out of the way of traffic and other people (skating rinks are great places to skate).

How To Play

If you're just beginning inline skating, here are some tips to get you rolling.

Practice balancing on your skates by walking in them on a flat, grassy area. As you move to the pavement, balance yourself without trying to move. Gradually begin to skate by moving forward, but not too fast. Keep your knees bent and flexible when you skate—it will keep you more stable. And if you fall—fall forward. Then you will fall on your kneepads—they're there to protect you!

It's also a good idea to take lessons from a certified instructor—you can find one through the International Inline Skating Association. As you get more skilled on your skates, there are several types of competitive inline skating activities—like speed skating and aggressive skating, which includes events like those at the X Games. There are also sports leagues just for those who play on wheels, such as roller hockey, roller soccer, and roller basketball.

Games

- Skate on one foot. Practice balancing on one foot at a time while you're skating. See how long you can glide on each foot. This is a great way to work on your balance!
- Skate with friends. Go inline skating at the local park or skating rink, or join a skate club in your town.
- Combine activities. Tired of just skating around in circles? Grab some friends for a game of inline hockey, inline basketball, or even inline soccer.

Skateboarding

Have you ever seen someone skateboarding and wanted to try it?

Gear Up

Skateboards can be bought preassembled, or you can buy all of the pieces and put it together yourself. Preassembled boards are best for beginners, until you decide if skateboarding is really for you. If you are putting your own board together, you'll need a deck (the board itself), grip tape for the top of the deck so your feet don't slip, 2 trucks (the metal parts that are the axles of the wheels), 4 wheels, and 2 bearings per wheel (these keep the wheels spinning on the truck's axle). Before each time you ride, make sure your trucks are tightened and your wheels are spinning properly. Don't forget to wear a helmet, knee and elbow pads, and wrist guards. It's important that your helmet is approved by one of the groups who test helmets to see which ones are the best: the Snell B-95 standard is best for skateboarding helmets. Nonslippery shoes are a good idea too, so you can have better control of your board.

Play It Safe

Before you ride, make sure you give your board a safety check to make sure everything is put together right. Always wear all of your protective gear including a helmet, knee and elbow pads, and wrist guards. If you do tricks with your board, you may also want to wear gloves to protect your hands from the pavement. If you're just starting out, skate on a smooth, flat surface so you can practice keeping control of your board. And no matter how experienced you are—never hold on to the back of a moving vehicle! It's best to skate out of the way of traffic and other people (skate parks are great places to skate). But if you are skating in streets near your house, be aware of cars and people around you, and stay out of their way. Also, once the sun sets, it's a good idea to put up your board for the night, since skating in the dark can be dangerous.

How To Play

If you're just starting out, follow these steps to develop your skateboarding skills. Put one foot on the board, toward the front, with the other on the ground. Push off the ground with your foot and put it on the rear of the board while you glide. Push again when you slow down.

There are several different styles of skateboarding:

- Street skating is skateboarding on streets, curbs, benches and handrails—anything involving common street objects. Street skating is best left to the pros though—it's very dangerous.
- Downhill skating is racing down big hills, usually on a longer skateboard called a longboard.
- Freestyle skating is more artistic, involving a series of tricks and stunts.
- Vert skating is skateboarding on mini-ramps and half pipes, which are U-shaped ramps.

If you start going too fast, step off the board with your back foot. To turn, shift your weight to your back foot so that the front truck lifts off the ground and then move your body in the direction you want to go—the board will go with you.

If you want to find half pipes, vert ramps, and skate courses near you to practice your moves, look for a nearby skate park, designed to give skateboarders a great ride.

Chapter 37

Soccer

Just what does it take to become a soccer All-star?

Gear Up

A ball. Soccer balls come in different sizes depending on how old you are. Kids 8-12 should use a size 4 ball, and kids 13 and over should use a size 5 ball. Synthetic leather balls are best for beginners, because they don't absorb water and get heavy.

If you play in a league, a goal will usually be provided for you, and you can buy a smaller goal if you want to play in your backyard—just make sure it is anchored to the ground. No goal? No problem! Just set up any two objects (cones or water bottles are good) to shoot between.

Two pieces of equipment you need to wear at all times when playing soccer are shin guards and cleats. Shin guards are designed to protect your legs from the ball, and from being kicked by other players. They are required in most leagues. The right cleats to wear for soccer are ones that are plastic or rubber—they'll help you with your quick starts, stops and turns.

Play It Safe

Be sure to wear shin guards and appropriate soccer cleats during games as well as practices. Warming up, especially your leg muscles, is very important. To avoid headaches and dizziness, use your head and learn the proper technique for heading a ball in a game. Many leagues have strict rules about wearing jewelry, watches, and barrettes during games. Since any of these items can cause you to get hurt if you're hit with a ball, it's a good idea to not wear them when you play. Also, to protect your mouth from collisions (especially if you have braces), wear a mouthguard.

About This Chapter: This chapter includes text excerpted from "BAM! Body And Mind—Soccer Activity Card," Centers for Disease Control and Prevention (CDC), May 9, 2015.

How To Play

In addition to a good strong kick, you'll want to master basic skills like passing (moving the ball to a teammate with a controlled kick), dribbling (tapping the ball with your feet to move it down the field), trapping (stopping the ball with your feet, legs, or chest), and heading (using your head to stop or pass the ball). Once you get these skills down, you'll be unstoppable!

Here are some great passing and trapping tips.

- **Passing.** Pick your target out before you start the pass. Keep your head down to make sure you kick the ball correctly. Plant your non-kicking foot next to the ball and kick the ball right in the center using the inside of your foot and follow through with your leg.

- **Chest trap.** As the ball comes toward you, get in front of it and let it hit your chest. Bring your shoulders around and slightly inward, creating a cavity for the ball. Make sure you keep your arms down, so the ball doesn't accidentally hit your hands and cause a foul. When the ball hits your chest, arch your back, so your chest pops the ball upward and then lands at your feet.

Ology

If you played soccer on top of a mountain, you'd be able to kick the ball much further. Why? The air pressure on top of a mountain is lower than at the bottom. When a soccer ball is kicked into the air, the air pressure pushes against the ball and slows it down. Since the air pressure on top of a mountain is much lower, there is less pressure to push against the ball and slow it down. As a result, the ball will go further.

Chapter 38

Tennis, Table Tennis, And Volleyball

Tennis

Want to know how to be a tennis all-star?

Gear Up

What's all the racket about racquets? Well, you can't play tennis without one. If you're buying a junior racquet, choose the longest one that you can comfortably use. Want more information on selecting a junior racquet? If you weigh more than 85 pounds you should look for an adult racquet.

When you have a racquet, you'll need to find a court. Look around at school or at parks in your neighborhood. Then, put on socks (if they're not cotton, they'll help you avoid blisters) and sneakers with good ankle support. Don't forget the tennis balls!

Games
- **Fish in the Pond:** Try tossing the ball onto your racquet or into a hula-hoop on the ground to practice aiming your toss.
- **Overhead Ball Catch:** Toss the ball up like you are about to serve and catch it just above your head.

About This Chapter: Text under the heading "Tennis" is excerpted from "BAM! Body And Mind—Tennis Activity Card," Centers for Disease Control and Prevention (CDC), May 9, 2015; Text under the heading "Table Tennis" is excerpted from "BAM! Body And Mind—Table Tennis Activity Card," Centers for Disease Control and Prevention (CDC), May 9, 2015; Text under the heading "Volleyball" is excerpted from "BAM! Body And Mind—Volleyball Activity Card," Centers for Disease Control and Prevention (CDC), May 9, 2015.

> • **Two-Handed Alligator Catch:** Stretch out your arms straight in front of you like they are the top and bottom of an alligator's mouth. Have a friend throw the ball toward you and slap your hands together to catch it. After each catch, make the alligator's mouth a little bigger.

Play It Safe

Tennis is an activity that forces you to turn your body quickly in many different directions, so make sure you warm up and stretch before playing. Wear tennis shoes with good support to protect your ankles and thick (not cotton) socks that fit well to prevent blisters on your feet. To prevent hand blisters, keep your racquet handle dry by using sawdust or hand chalk. Always bend your arm when you swing, or else it might start to hurt—a problem known as "tennis elbow." Clip your toenails and make sure there is extra room in your shoes, because "tennis toe" can be nasty too!

To protect other players, never throw your racquet or tennis balls, and try to keep loose balls off the courts. Be courteous and keep yourself and others safe by staying off courts where other people are playing.

When you're outside waiting to play, sit in the shade and drink lots of water—that way you'll stay cool and won't get sunburned. While you are playing, take a break between games or sets to cool off. And you may want to keep a wet towel around your neck while you wait. Also, you can look and feel cool by wearing a cold, wet bandana on your head while you play. And always wear sunscreen!

How To Play

Tennis is a fun activity that two people (a "singles" match) or four people on two separate teams ("doubles") can play. You can play with friends at your local tennis courts, or join an organized team. When you start playing tennis, some of the keystrokes you should learn are: serve, forehand, backhand, two-handed backhand, volley, and smash. But first, check out these basic skills to get you started!

Holding the Racquet. The racquet handle has eight sides—four are flat and four are angled. Take the racquet handle between your thumb and index finger of your dominant hand (the one you write with) as if you were shaking hands. The knuckle on your index finger should be on the top right angle. Then, grip and make sure it feels comfortable. Separate your third and fourth fingers slightly.

Serving. Hold the ball with the thumb, index finger, and middle finger of your free hand (hand not holding the racquet). Extend the arm with the ball just in front of you and then raise it above your head. Toss the ball gently, so it goes a few inches higher than the full height of the racquet extended above your head. Keep your eye on the ball. Bring the racquet around above your shoulder and hit the ball while it's in the air. Try to use the same toss every time.

Receiving and Returning the Ball. Stand in the middle of the court and hold the racquet gently with both hands so you can run in either direction when the ball comes over the net. When the ball is hit to your forehand side (e.g., right if you're right-handed), step toward the ball with your opposite leg and swing! If the ball comes to your backhand side (left if you're right-handed), go for the ball with your dominant arm in front of your chest and your other hand holding the racquet as well. Swing without moving your wrists.

Ology

Wondering why tennis balls are so fuzzy? The fuzz increases the wind resistance, which slows down the ball and helps the players to volley (hit the ball back and forth without stopping) longer. Without it, the ball would fly off the court after every serve! The fuzz also helps players control the ball, by keeping it stuck to their racquet strings for just a little longer when they hit it.

Table Tennis

Table tennis is a fun indoor game.

Gear Up

You'll need the right equipment to get started. First, you'll want a table. The tables that are used look a lot like a tennis court—they are usually rectangular and green with white lines. A six-inch net is used to divide the table in half.

Next, you'll need a ball and paddles. The balls used in tournaments and during professional competitions are made of plastic and are hollow inside. Paddles, sometimes called rackets, are mostly made of wood. Each side is covered with a sheet of rubber. Often times the rubber sheets are made with different textures. This allows players to hit the ball at different speeds and with different types of spin. Even if a player chose different textures for each side of the paddle, official regulations require one side to be red and one side to be black. This way, players can always tell which side of the paddle their opponent is using.

Games

Chances are, you've played table tennis at school or at a friend's house. But did you know table tennis, also called Ping-Pong, is one of the most popular competitive sports in the world? It can be very different from what you might play at school or at home with friends. Table tennis is played at a very fast pace—some people even say it's the fastest ball sport in the world! This makes it really challenging and requires athletes to be in great shape. AND, they have to have super hand-eye coordination!

Table tennis is a pretty new when you compare it to sports like running or soccer. In fact, it started at the end of the 19th century. It's believed that table tennis began in England where people used common household objects like corks and box lids to play. Once hollow, plastic balls replaced the cork and rubber balls originally used, the game became popular in North America too. These new balls allowed people to play with more bounce and at a much faster pace which helped to turn the game into a competitive sport.

Play It Safe

During any physical activity, it's always important to play it safe! Understanding the rules of a game always helps, and you should do things like stretching to help prevent injuries. So when playing table tennis, make sure you play by the rules and stay alert. It's also a good idea to rest in between training sessions so that your body can relax and your muscles can recover from the workout!

How To Play

First, you'll need to know how to stand and hold your paddle. Hold your arm out in front of you—like you're about to shake hands. Then extend your fingers but keep your thumb pointing up. The paddle's handle should rest between your thumb and forefinger, and its face should point up like your thumb. Close your fingers around the handle, and use your forefinger and thumb for control. You'll want to grip the handle firmly, but keep it relaxed. Simply tighten your grip for more powerful shots.

Stand far enough from the table so that your arm and paddle can be fully extended. Shift your weight to the balls of your feet, and keep your knees slightly bent. Lean forward a bit, using your non-paddle hand to keep balance.

Toss the ball up for a serve, and let it bounce one time before hitting it. Each player serves five times, and then the serve goes to their opponent.

Stand like you're about to serve the ball for a forehand shot. Only this time, face sideways so that your non-paddle shoulder points toward the other player. Swing your paddle back, shifting your hips in the same direction. Remember that the further you swing back, the more powerful the shot will be. Hold the paddle at the height of your waist, and keep your wrist tilted slightly toward the floor. This way you'll hit the ball in an upward direction and send it over the net. Swing your arms and hips forward, and take your shot!

When you take a backhand shot, your thumb should be on the back of your paddle. Like in the forehand shot, your non-paddle shoulder should face your opponent, and the paddle should be waist-high. Let your elbow lead your arm as you swing quickly and hit the ball as it bounces off the table.

Scoring

There are a variety of ways to score a point. You'll score when a server makes a bad serve or when a player isn't able to hit the ball back to the other player. Points are also scored if the ball bounces two or more times on one player's side, or if the player touches the net or table.

Volleyball

Want to be a volleyball player all-star?

Gear Up

A ball. Volleyballs are about 26 inches around and weigh a bit more than half a pound.

A net. The net is stretched across the middle of the court and adjusts to different heights—7 1/2 feet for girls and 8 feet for guys.

Elbow and knee pads. When you're playing volleyball, you're probably going to hit the ground a few times. Protect yourself with pads.

Volleyball shoes. The bottoms of volleyball shoes are made of special rubber to keep you from slipping as you move around the court. Your shoes should also give you good ankle support and have lots of cushioning to protect your feet while you're jumping.

Play It Safe

Be sure to wear knee and elbow pads when you're playing on a hard court to protect you when you dive for the ball. When you go up for the ball, try landing on the balls of your feet with your knees bent and your hips lowered a little. Also, warm up and stretch before you play, and take off any jewelry.

Communicate with your teammates while you're playing to keep from running into each other. Make sure everyone on the team knows to "call" the ball by saying "got it" or "mine" if they plan to go for it.

If you're playing outside, find a soft court made of sand or grass, and clean up any sharp objects that you see. Be sure that there aren't any trees or basketball hoops in your way. And, wear sunscreen and always drink plenty of water. If you're playing inside, the court should be made of wood.

If your volleyball net is held up by wires, make sure they are covered with soft materials. That way you won't get hurt if you accidentally jump or run into the net.

How To Play

Volleyball is fun to play because everybody gets involved! The game is unique because the same player isn't allowed to hit the ball twice in a row, so everyone takes turns serving, passing, and setting the ball. A team can hit the ball up to three times before they get it over the net. Before you play, check out these moves!

- **Serving the ball.** Stand at the back of the court and face the net. Hold the ball in the palm of your non-dominant hand (for example, left if you're right-handed) and stretch out your arm at waist level. Lean forward and swing your dominant hand (the one you write with) up toward the bottom of the ball. Now, drop the ball and hit it with your fist or the bottom of your hitting hand. Follow through, pointing your hitting arm toward your target. Finally, get ready to score. Only the team that's serving can score points! After you have practiced this underhand for a while, you can try a powerful overhead serve!

- **Passing the ball.** Move to the place where you think the ball will land and stand with your feet shoulder-width apart. Bend your knees and put your arms straight out in front of you. Lock your hands together with your thumbs pointed forward. Watch the ball make contact with your arms and then push it forward with your forearms. Aim with your shoulders and straighten your legs, using the force from your legs to move the ball where you want it to go.

- **Setting the ball.** Stand with your feet shoulder-width apart, facing your target. Bend your knees and raise your hands above your head with your elbows bent. Put your hands together about six inches above and in front of your forehead, and make a diamond shape with your thumbs and pointer fingers. When the ball comes to you, use only your thumbs and the tops of your fingers to push the ball up in the direction you want it to go. Your palms should not touch the ball.

Ology

Volleyball is all about physics! The force of the volleyball hitting your arms is the action, and the force of you hitting the ball is the reaction. If these forces were equal, you wouldn't be able to move the ball off your arms. But since the force of you pushing the ball is stronger than the force of the ball pushing into you, you're able to change the ball's direction and pass it to your teammate. If the ball's force ever became stronger than your own, it would knock you to the ground.

Chapter 39

Walking And Hiking

Walking

Walking means more than transportation.

Gear Up

Shoes are the most important part of your walking gear. Good walking shoes are generally flat, but flexible, so your foot rolls with each step. They should fit well, but leave enough room for your feet to spread out while walking. Wear socks that are comfortable. Try socks made of cotton or other sweat-wicking materials—they will keep your feet drier and help prevent blisters. Running shoes are okay to use for walking. Don't forget to trade in the old shoes when the treads start wearing out—which is about 500 miles.

Wear comfortable clothing when walking. Try to dress in layers, so you can always take off something as you warm up. Layering with a t-shirt, sweatshirt, or windproof jacket is a good idea if it's windy or chilly outside.

Two other essentials: sunscreen and a hat. The sunscreen protects your skin from the sun. In the summer, a hat keeps the sun out of your face, and in the winter it helps to keep you warm by trapping the heat that is lost from the top of your head. A bright colored hat will also make it easy for drivers to see and avoid you.

About This Chapter: Text under the heading "Walking" is excerpted from "BAM! Body And Mind—Walking Activity Card," Centers for Disease Control and Prevention (CDC), May 9, 2015; Text under the heading "Hiking" is excerpted from "BAM! Body And Mind—Hiking Activity Card," Centers for Disease Control and Prevention (CDC), May 9, 2015.

Play It Safe

Before you walk out the door, talk about the best walking routes with your parents so you know your safety zones and how to avoid traffic. And, only walk in those areas so your parents will know where you are.

It's always best to walk where you can avoid traffic—like parks or even the mall! Or try to find an area where there are sidewalks. If you have to walk on a street without sidewalks, walk close to the curb facing traffic. Remember to cross the street only at marked crosswalks or at corners, keep your ears and eyes open, and watch out for traffic in front and back of you. Wear bright-colored clothing or reflectors so drivers can see you. If you are walking alone, don't wear headphones—if they are too loud, they can keep you from hearing any oncoming traffic.

It's a good idea to drink some water before you head out to walk, while you are walking, and when you get back—even if it's cold outside or you don't feel thirsty. In the summer, late afternoons (not nights) and mornings are the best times to walk to avoid the midday heat and humidity.

It is best to warm up your muscles before stretching them. So warm up for 5 minutes at an easy walking pace before stretching. Then stretch by starting at the top of your body and working your way down. Make sure to cool down and stretch after your walk too!

Remember—start out slowly and gradually increase the speed and distance you walk—don't try walking a marathon your first time out! And no matter where you are walking, be aware of what is going on around you.

How To Play

You've probably been walking for about as long as you've been talking. But walking isn't just a way to get from here to there, its also a great physical activity! Walking doesn't require a lot of equipment, you can do it anywhere, it is always available by just walking out your front door, and it's a great way to relax and refresh. It's also something you can do alone or with your friends and family.

If you thought walking was just putting one foot in front of the other, you were right! But check out these tips for how to walk and breathe correctly so your walk will be safer and easier.

Posture. How you hold your body is important. Stand up straight and tall. This means putting your shoulders back and relaxing them (no slouching!), and keeping your chin up and stomach in. It's a good idea to look 20 feet ahead—about the lengths of two cars. This keeps your chin up and your eyes on your path!

Taking your first steps. Start out your first step with the heel first. Then roll your foot from heel to toe and push off the toes with the next step. Bringing the opposite leg forward, repeat this again. (This may feel a little funny at first but as your muscles get stronger it gets easier.)

Arm motion. Moving or swinging your arms when you're walking can give you power and it balances what your legs are doing! Bend your elbow 90 degrees (so your arm looks like the letter "L"), while keeping your hands slightly curled. When you step, one foot moves forward and the arm opposite this foot should come forward too. As your foot goes back, bring back the opposite arm with it. Keep your elbows close to the body so you don't have "chicken wings."

Don't forget to breathe! Your breathing should have a rhythm. Inhale one deep breath for four steps and then hold that breath for two steps. Then exhale to the count of four steps, and hold it for two steps before beginning all over again. So the rhythm is—breathe in (step 1, 2, 3, 4), hold (step 1, 2) breathe out (step 1, 2, 3, 4) hold (step 1, 2).

Everyone's stride is different, so if you feel that four steps are too long or too short, adjust it to what is comfortable for you.

Ology

We don't give a second thought to walking and breathing at the same time, but some ancient creatures, and some that are still around (like lizards), can't do both at once. Lizards have to pause when they're running in order to take breaths.

Hiking

Take a hike! No, really, take the time to go hiking.

Gear Up

First, you'll need a good pair of shoes and thick socks designed for this type of activity. You can start with some sturdy sneakers with thick bottoms. When you begin to take on more difficult trails, try a pair of hiking boots, and make sure they fit! Also, get a backpack or fanny pack to carry all of your hiking supplies. Dress in layers and bring along a waterproof jacket with a hood in case you get caught in the rain. And don't forget a hat, sunscreen, and sunglasses because the higher you hike, the more dangerous the sun's rays become.

To keep hiking fun, you always need to be prepared to beat problems that could happen while you're out, like finding the trail if you get lost or stuck in bad weather. Make sure you bring a map of the area you'll be hiking in and a sturdy compass. Don't know how to use a compass? Check this out to learn how. You'll also need to bring plenty of water and extra food, like sports bars or trail mix, in case you have to stay out late and get hungry. The adults on your hike should bring a box of waterproof matches and an Army-style knife. A flashlight and extra batteries will help you find your way if you end up out after dark. Finally, you'll need to bring a first aid kit, in case someone gets hurt during your hike.

Play It Safe

Prep. Get in shape before you head out on your hike. Try walking around your neighborhood with your pack loaded with five pounds more gear than you'll actually carry on your hike. If that goes well, plan a short hike to test your abilities on the trail.

Buddies. Take a friend and an adult along on your hike. That way you can look out for each other and you'll have people to talk to! Also, be sure to let someone who's not going know where you'll be hiking and what time you'll be back.

H_2O. Carry lots of water even if you are only planning a short hike. For warm-weather hikes, bring six to eight quarts of water per day. In the cold weather or higher elevations, you can be safe with half that amount. Whenever you are near water, make sure you wet yourself down. Dampen a bandana and wipe your face, neck, and arms or wrap it around your head while you hike.

Blisters and more. To prevent blisters, try spraying your feet with an antiperspirant before heading out. Bring extra pairs of socks that you can change into if your feet get wet or sweaty—if they aren't made of cotton, they'll keep your feet drier. Once you're on the trail, stop as soon as you feel a "hot spot" on your feet and apply special type of bandage called "moleskin" to the sore area. Also, try using a hiking stick to keep some pressure off of your legs and knees.

Buzz. Don't get bugged by bugs. Protect yourself from bites and stings by using a bug repellant that includes (Diethyl-meta-toluamide) DEET. Repellents that contain DEET are the most effective, but make sure you rub them on according to the directions. A good rule of thumb from the experts is that kids should use repellents with less than 10 percent DEET. Get your parents to help you put it on your face so you don't get it in your mouth or eyes. And wash your hands after you apply it. Remember that stuff that smells good to you smells good to bugs too, so don't use scented shampoos or lotions before hiking.

Weather watcher. When it's hot, pick trails that are shaded and run near streams. If you need to hike uphill in the sun, first soak yourself down to stay cool. You can also try wearing a wet bandana around your head or neck. Also, try to stay out of cotton clothes. Keep yourself out of bad weather by checking forecasts before you hike and watching the skies once you're out on the trail. During lightning storms, head downhill and away from the direction of the storm, and then squat down and keep your head low.

Keep it yummy. To stay healthy on your hike, you'll need to know how to keep your food and water safe. Remember the four C's: contain, clean, cook, and chill.

How To Play

Hiking with your friends or family is a great chance to get outdoors, breathe some fresh air, and get active. It's easy to get started. Just look for a trail in a national park near you!

For your first day hike (hiking for a day or less without camping overnight), choose a safe, well-marked trail that doesn't have too many steep climbs. Otherwise, you'll get tired too early and won't make it as far as you want to go. Each time you go hiking, try going a little farther and take a slightly steeper trail. Before you know it you'll be hiking the Appalachian Trail—a 2,167-mile trail that goes all the way from Maine to Georgia!

Chapter 40

Water Sports

Canoeing/Kayaking

Just what does it take to canoe or kayak?

Gear Up

You'll need a kayak (boat that's almost completely closed on top with space for just one person) or a canoe (open boat that can fit you and a friend or two) plus the right kind of paddle. Kayak paddles have a blade on both sides, but canoe paddles have one blade. Be sure to pick the right size paddle—the stick part of a canoe paddle should be about six to eight inches longer than the length of your arm with your fingers out. Don't forget another essential: the life vest! Water shoes or sneakers—not sandals—that grip on the bottom will help your feet stay put when you are pulling the paddle through the water. Keep a whistle attached to your life vest so you are always ready to get attention if trouble strikes.

About This Chapter: Text under the heading "Canoeing/Kayaking" is excerpted from "BAM! Body And Mind—Canoeing/Kayaking Activity Card," Centers for Disease Control and Prevention (CDC), May 9, 2015; Text under the heading "Diving" is excerpted from "BAM! Body And Mind—Diving Activity Card," Centers for Disease Control and Prevention (CDC), May 9, 2015; Text under the heading "Snorkel" is excerpted from "BAM! Body And Mind—Snorkeling Activity Card," Centers for Disease Control and Prevention (CDC), May 9, 2015; Text under the heading "Surfing" is excerpted from "BAM! Body And Mind—Surfing Activity Card," Centers for Disease Control and Prevention (CDC), May 9, 2015; Text under the heading "Water Skiing" is excerpted from "BAM! Body And Mind—Water Skiing Activity Card," Centers for Disease Control and Prevention (CDC), May 9, 2015; Text under the heading "White-Water Rafting" is excerpted from "BAM! Body And Mind—White-Water Rafting Activity Card," Centers for Disease Control and Prevention (CDC), May 9, 2015.

Play It Safe

You need to be a strong swimmer because you might have to swim underwater, or in moving water. Always go paddling with another person—not just for times of trouble, but because someone should help you carry, load, and launch your boat, right?

Make sure your life jacket fits. Since paddling is an activity that you can do all through the year, leave enough room to put clothes under it when it is cold out. Be prepared to get wet! Take along extra dry clothing, just in case. Remember to keep sun proof with sunscreen.

Save paddling for good weather days. Since you don't know what Mother Nature will throw at you, know where your float trip will take you, spots where you can get out or camp for the night, and different ways to go in case unexpected trouble strikes your route. Avoid whitewater rapids, dams, and falls—only experienced whitewater paddlers should take these on.

Sure, you want all your friends and their stuff to come along, but don't put too much weight in the boat—you should have more than six inches of side between the top of the fully loaded boat and the water. Spread out the weight (including people) so the boat will stay balanced.

Take lessons to help you learn ways to get yourself back in your boat if it tips over—before you take your first trip. And then practice them. The main thing to remember is—Don't panic. If you can't get back in, stay with your boat and flip it back over—it'll float—and try to swim the boat to shore.

How To Play

Canoeing. Hold the paddle with your inside hand on top and your water-side hand two to three feet down. Your knuckles should be facing out. Without stretching, insert the blade of the paddle all the way in the water as far forward as you can reach. Push your top hand forward and pull your bottom hand back, turning your shoulders to move the paddle blade straight through the water to your hip. Keep the top of the paddle handle lower than your eyes and don't follow the curve of the canoe. Again! Have a friend paddle on the other side of the canoe, or switch sides as you paddle, to keep the boat gliding along straight.

Kayaking. Kayak paddles have a blade on each side. Lift your paddle with both hands and hold it across your chest. Place your hands the same distance from each blade, just outside your shoulders. Hold the paddle out in front of you, just a few inches above the kayak. Keeping your left elbow straight, bring your right hand straight back, letting your right elbow bend back toward your body. Your body will twist to the right a bit. Paddle. Now, use the other arm. You're kayaking!

Kayakers and canoers follow these tips so they don't annoy other people—or the environment!

Ology

A Greek mathematician named Archimedes figured out that when something is in water, the force that keeps it afloat is equal to the weight of the water that it pushes aside. Light objects (like a leaf) float because they push aside more than their own weight in water, but heavy objects (like a rock) sink because they push aside less than their own weight. A canoe pushes aside more water that its weight, which means it can carry heavy stuff inside and still float.

Diving

Just what does it take to become a diver?

Gear Up

It's simple—all you need is a swimsuit and a pool with a diving board. Check out your neighborhood or a community center in your area for a pool you can use.

Play It Safe

Here's the deal: Know how to swim well before stepping on the board. Always dive with someone else. And… Protect your noggin! You've gotta know the water depth before you dive, and never ever dive into shallow water. Check around for signs or ask a lifeguard. Diving areas are usually marked. In case you haven't figured this out yet, above-ground pools are not designed for diving. They're way too shallow! (Lots of in-ground pools aren't deep enough either, so check out the water before you dive.)

When you are on the board, enter the water straight on and make sure there's nothing in your way before you leap. If people come into the diving area from other parts of the pool, wait until they're gone, or just ask the lifeguard to clear the area for you. If you jump when there is someone else in the diving area, or even just mess around while diving, you could land on top of someone and get hurt!

Don't run up to a dive. Always stand at the edge of the board or pool and then dive. And dive straight ahead—not off to the side.

It's also important to warm-up and stretch before diving, and then cool down after your plunge session.

Most of all, only try dives that are in your comfort zone. Leave those fancy or stunt leaps to experienced divers. An adult can help you decide which dives are safe to try.

How To Play

Diving is about precision, flexibility, and strength—all in one! Experienced divers leap 5-10 meters (about 16-33 feet) into the air from a springboard or platform, do stunts like somersaults or twists, and then plunge into the water below.

Be water wise. Check the depth before you dive.

A certified diving instructor can help you master the diving board, but for now, try this beginners' dive—Point your arms straight over your head, with your shoulders by your ears. Keep your head between your arms and tuck your chin to your chest. Bend at the waist, but don't bend the knees. Keep your legs straight. Fall towards the water, making sure not to lift your head or shoulders. Follow through with your fingers into the water. That's it—you've made the plunge!

Ology

How can a diver flip and twist so fast in the air before hitting the water? To find out, try this experiment: Sit in a chair that spins and have a friend turn you. When your friend moves away from the chair, tuck your arms and legs in close to your chest. Notice that you will start to spin much faster. This shows how divers can spin faster when they suddenly draw their arms inward (tuck position). If your arms were stretched out, you wouldn't move as fast because the resistance of the air would slow you down. But if your arms are tucked beside you, there is less resistance and your body spins faster.

Snorkeling

Snorkeling is just like swimming, but with fins, a mask, and a tube called a snorkel for breathing underwater.

Gear Up

To snorkel you don't need a lot of complicated equipment—a mask, snorkel, fins, and swimsuit or swimming trunks are all you need.

Mask. It's important to buy a good mask that's the right size for your face and has a tight-fitting seal. The easiest way to test how well your mask fits is to lift the strap over the top of the mask and press the mask to your face without breathing in. If it stays tight to your face (without you holding it on), you've got the right fit. If not, keep looking until you find one that seals properly. You'll want to get a mask that has a glass face (not plastic) to keep it from fogging up or making the sites below look weird.

Snorkel. There are many different sizes and designs of snorkels—find one that is comfortable, and allows you to clear water easily. It's important that you find the right snorkel for you—it's what helps you breathe while you're cruising along in the water checking out the sites below.

Fins. There are a few different types of fins to choose from—full-foot fins fit like a slipper around your heel, while open-heel fins fit your feet and have a strap that fits around your heel. Your fins should be snug, but not too tight (if your fins are too tight or loose, they may cause blisters). They should be flexible and lightweight—to give you speed and mobility. You may also want to get diving booties to prevent blisters and protect our feet.

If you're swimming in salty water, make sure to rinse all of your equipment with fresh water. If you don't, salt crystals can form causing the straps to stiffen and crack, and the fabric may tear. So, keep your equipment clean. Remember, it's what allows you to move through the water and check out the underwater world more easily!

Play It Safe

Always make sure your snorkel, fins, and mask are in good working order before taking the plunge. It's also important to know the basics like how to clear water from your snorkel (blasting), and how to put your mask back on while treading water. Until you get more experienced, you may want to wear a life jacket—it will help you stay afloat if you need a rest, or if you get into trouble in the water.

Most importantly, never snorkel alone. Always swim with a buddy and keep them close by so you can help each other out—and, it's more fun with a friend!

Use your noggin'—check out the weather forecast and the water's visibility before you jump in. And don't forget, coral reefs are fun to explore, but don't go too close to them until you've learned how to steer your body in the water. Never touch a reef—they are sharp and some have ocean life that may be poisonous. Always be considerate of the places you are snorkeling in, they may be another animal's home.

Finally, watch out for the sun! Wear a t-shirt and sunscreen to make sure you don't get sunburned.

How To Play

Before heading out to explore the water, it's important to know how to swim. Finding the right mask or snorkel should be next on your list.

Learning to use a snorkel is easy. You may want to practice in a swimming pool (or shallow water where you can stand) until you get the hang of it. First, put your mask on—it should have a small rubber strap that attaches the snorkel to your mask, and the snorkel should pass just above your left ear. Take a deep breath, bite down on the mouthpiece and slowly place your head into the water (make sure to breathe through your mouth). Breathe out through your mouth once to clear any water out of the snorkel—this is called blasting. Inhale slowly in case there's water in your tube, then blast your snorkel again just to make sure you get as much water out as you can. Swim along the surface of the water at a slow pace. If you swim too fast, or make lots of sudden movements with your arms and legs, you can scare the fish and other sea creatures away!

After you get the hang of using your snorkel and mask, you may want to take a dive. Try some shallow dives to get an idea of how long you can hold your breath. It's important to know your limits.

Ology

Ever wonder why your ears pop when you dive down into the deep end of a swimming pool, or when you're swimming in the ocean and go under too far? Well, it has to do with pressure—both from the water pushing in on you, and the air trapped in your ears pushing out.

To solve the problem of pressure in your ears, you can even it out by holding your nose shut with your fingers and blowing into your nose. You will hear your ears pop and the pain and pressure should go away. If this doesn't work, try yawning—this trick also helps to release the pressure.

Surfing

Do you live close to the coast and beach? This is a sport that uses waves.

Gear Up

All you really need is a bathing suit or a wetsuit (for cold water or if it's cold out), and of course, a surfboard!

Here are some tips:

You may want to get a used or inexpensive board at first. It wouldn't be smart to mess up a cool, new board making beginner's mistakes. The fins should be in good condition, and it should have a place to attach a leash (cord that hooks your ankle to the board so it doesn't get away). Long boards are easier to ride and control. Your board should be 12 to 14 inches taller than you. Also, put two coats of wax on your board if the deck (top) doesn't have a pad that keeps you from slipping.

Play It Safe

What do surfing and walking a dog have in common? Well, surfboards don't bark, but they still need a "leash" to keep them from getting away! Surfing takes lots of practice, but when you're riding that wave, it's incredible! Here's how to start:

- **Goofy Foot?** Put your best foot forward—find out whether you are regular or goofy-footed! Try sliding across a smooth floor with socks on. If you lead with your left foot, you're "regular," and the left foot goes near the front of the board when you're surfing. If your right foot goes first, you're "goofy," and the right foot goes up front!

- **Paddling.** To get around in the water, lay chest-down on your board, keeping your legs straight behind you. With each arm, make an overhand swimming stroke that starts at the front of the board and finishes under the board near your legs. (It's like swimming the crawl stroke, except you're on top of the board!) As you finish the stroke with one hand, the other hand is just starting. Try practicing in shallow water or a pool first.

- **Catching the Wave.** When you see white water (breaking waves) coming, turn around to face the shore, aim your board the direction the wave is coming, and start to paddle in. When the wave reaches you, it will push you forward. Stop paddling, grab the side of the board, push up your body, and quickly get your feet under you. Both should land at the same time, toes pointing sideways. Move your lead (regular or goofy) foot in front. Hey, you're surfing!

How To Play

First things first—You've gotta be a strong swimmer. As a beginner, you are going to be in the water more than riding your board! And always surf with someone else.

While you're a beginner, stick to waves no bigger than three feet. If you are a real beginner, surf only broken (white) waves. Never paddle out farther than you can swim back with your board. Most of all, if it doesn't feel right or you are too scared, just don't go!

Always leash your board to control it. When you begin the wipeout (fall at the end of a ride), kick your board out and away from you.

Bad weather = No surfing.

Did you know that surfers have rules for who "owns" a wave? Surfers riding waves have to get out of the way of those paddling out, and everyone has to stay clear of swimmers. A surfer who is standing and riding a wave gets to keep it—no one should "drop in" (try to catch the same wave). Finally, make sure to wear sunscreen.

Ology

Everything has the potential to move, known as potential energy. When it does move, it changes into kinetic (moving) energy. A wave is potential energy that travels a very far distance across the water. This energy is created by stuff like the wind. When the potential energy in the water changes into kinetic energy, the water starts moving, making waves. Surfers catch a small bit of this force, jump on their boards, get up, and surf.

Water Skiing

When you think of water skiing, do you think of a lazy afternoon at the lake — a boat pulling a skier behind it? Well, think again!

Gear Up

First you'll need water skis. There are four types: combination pairs, slalom, tick, and jump skis. New skiers should start with combination pairs, since they are wider and easiest to learn on. Make sure your skis have been checked and that they fit properly. You will also need a flexible towrope that has a floating handle.

All water skiers wear life vests (a.k.a. personal floatation devices or PFDs). You should wear a special water skiing life vest that is approved by the Coast Guard. You and your parents should check this out to get the official word on which life vest is right for you.

Play It Safe

Water skiers need to be good swimmers and always wear a life jacket that fits properly.

Safe water skiing requires three people: the skier, an experienced boat driver, and the spotter to look out for the skier's signals. Since the noise from the boat is so loud, it's important that everyone agrees on and understands the hand signals to use so you can talk without saying a word! Remember, you need to master hand signals before you begin cutting across the water on your skis!

When you're out on the water, be sure you're in a safe area to ski. Don't ski near docks, boats, rocks, or in shallow water. The only place to start is in the water—dock or land starts should be left to the pros.

If you start to lose your balance while skiing, just bend your knees and crouch down so you don't fall. If you do fall—and everyone does—remember to let go of the rope! Then, find your skis and hold one of them up to signal you're okay and to let other boaters know you're in the water.

How To Play

Want to walk on water? Try water skiing! Water skiers hold onto a rope and are pulled on their skis behind a boat going fast. They glide across the water with the wind in their faces! It's a great activity that you can do with your family or friends and it can be competitive. Check out these tips and you'll be skiing in no time!

Getting Started. Before you get in the water to ski, make sure you're wearing a life vest that is the right size and is on the right way. Get in the water with your skis. Wet your ski bindings before you put on your skis, and keep the bindings loose enough that the skis will come off if you fall. Bend your knees up towards your chest with your arms straight out in front of you. As the boat pulls the rope toward you, grab the rope handle with both hands and hold it between your knees. You should almost be sitting on the skis. Facing the boat, lift the tips of your skis a bit above the water, keep your skis shoulder width apart, and keep your arms straight. Nod your head to let the boat driver know you are ready to go, and begin straightening your legs as you are pulled out of the water. If you stand too soon you'll fall down, so take it slow and be patient.

Steering. To turn, just lean in the direction you want to go. Move your weight to the edge of the skis on the side you want to turn toward while you keep the skis pointed forward. If you want to turn faster, crouch down while you lean.

White-water rafting is an exciting way to see the great outdoors while testing your strength and ability to think on your feet.

White-Water Rafting

White-water rafting is an exciting way to see the great outdoors while testing your strength and ability to think on your feet.

Gear Up

You'll need a raft and paddles (usually 8 people per raft) to navigate the rapids, as well as a good life jacket and helmet. If you're heading out into cooler temperatures, wear warm, waterproof clothing and wool socks—these will keep you warm and dry while splashing down the river. If it's warm outside, nylon shorts, a bathing suit or swim trunks, a t-shirt, or a tank top are all good choices—just make sure to lather on that sunscreen to protect yourself from the sun. As for shoes, your best bet is to wear a pair with rubber soles or slip-on water shoes that you don't mind getting wet—because even during a good run, you're sure to get wet!

Some rafting trips can take a few hours (or even an entire day), so pack plenty of drinking water and food—just make sure to pack it up tight to keep the water out.

Play It Safe

Before jumping into that raft, it's important to know how to swim. Even if you're a strong swimmer, always wear a life jacket. It should fit snugly and have back and shoulder protection as well as floatation to help you swim safely in white water. Also, don't forget to wear your helmet—it should be designed for water sports, fit properly and snugly on your head, and allow for water to drain from the helmet. It should also cover your ears, temples, and the back of your neck. Once you have the proper gear and are sure it's all in working order, you're ready to run the river.

It's also really helpful if you've done a little exploring first. Make sure you know the river you are rafting on—check out the rating of the rapids and what the current is like. It's best to a have a trained, experienced guide on your team and in your raft. The guide will know the best course and the safest passage. Don't enter a rapid unless you're sure you can run it safely or swim it without getting hurt. If you fall out of the raft, position your body so that you are on your back with your feet facing down river—try to keep your feet and legs up.

Usually a group of three boats is the minimum on a river—but only one boat should run the rapids at a time. Safe rafting is all about teamwork, so pick a captain to call out directions so everyone can work together.

Most importantly, be prepared! Get a first aid and survival kit, and include extra ropes, a raft repair kit, and extra life vests. Better safe than stranded!

How To Play

White-water rafting is definitely a team effort—that's why understanding the basics of paddling are so important. If everyone in the raft gives it their all, it's much easier to guide the raft down the river and through the rapids.

Once you're in the raft, sit facing downriver with your back to the stern (back of the raft). Hold the paddle with your inside hand (the hand farthest away from the paddle) on top and your outside hand, knuckles facing out, gripping the paddle low on the stern. Lean forward from your hips, straighten your arms out in front of you, and keep your back straight. Straighten your wrists and put the paddle into the water—make sure the blade is completely under the surface of the water. Straighten your top arm while pulling back the paddle with your lower arm guiding the paddle. Reverse this motion to back paddle. If you want to turn the raft right, the right side of your rafting team needs to paddle backward while the left side paddles forward. The same goes for turning left except the members on the left side of the raft need to paddle backward and the right side forward. Rafting is all about communicating and working as a team!

Ology

Water is strange stuff—whether it's in a glass, frozen like an ice cube, or boiling on the stove, it's pretty much all the same, but when it starts to move, the physics of water becomes very complicated.

It's easy to see how powerful Mother Nature is when you watch rapids in a fast-flowing river. Water pounds against rocks, sprays into the sky, and boils into white foam. Rapids look chaotic, but really are predictable. The volume of water, the steepness (or gradient) of the river, the width of the channel, and the obstacles in the water all have effects on the rapids. The river's speed increases as more water flows through it—double the water means double the speed, so a mild rapid becomes a dangerous one during the rainy season. Rafters also must know the flow because water is heavy, and in rapids it exerts tremendous pressure on a raft.

Chapter 41

Winter Sports

Figure Skating

Just what does it take to become a figure skater?

Gear Up

Figure skates are very thick and heavy and have a toe pick attached for tricks. Figure skates are made up of two parts, the boot and the blade. If you are just starting out, you can buy skates with both a boot and a blade, but more advanced skaters can buy each separately. The boot should be snug in the heel and supportive of the ankle. The blade is attached to the boot with screws, and is wider than the blade on an ice hockey skate, so that the edge grips the ice. You should not use figure skates to play ice hockey, because the blades extend past the boot and can cause other players to get injured.

If you are a beginning skater, along with your skates, you may want to wear a helmet to protect your head against any falls.

Be sure to wear layers so that you can put on or take off clothes depending on whether you are cold or warm. It's important to be able to move, so sweatpants or warm-up pants are perfect. You should only wear one pair of lightweight socks inside your skates, though, and remember to wear mittens and a hat to keep warm.

About This Chapter: Text under the heading "Figure Skating" is excerpted from "BAM! Body And Mind—Figure Skating Activity Card," Centers for Disease Control and Prevention (CDC), May 9, 2015; Text under the heading "Snow Skiing" is excerpted from "BAM! Body And Mind—Snow Skiing Activity Card," Centers for Disease Control and Prevention (CDC), May 9, 2015.

Play It Safe

Be a courteous skater—always be aware of other skaters and follow the traffic flow of the rink. Be careful not to get too close to other skaters with your exposed blades. And keep your skate laces tied tightly so that you don't trip yourself or anyone else up.

If you feel yourself beginning to fall, bring your hands, arms, and head into your body to absorb the shock of hitting the ice. And make sure you hop up quickly so that you are not in the way of other skaters.

Skating can be hard work, and puts a lot of stress on your leg and back muscles, so be sure to warm-up before you skate and stretch those muscles well.

How To Play

Did you ever watch the figure skaters in the Olympics wondering how the heck they did all those jumps and spins? Well, according to the Xperts, the key to becoming a successful skater is one simple thing—balance. Good posture is an important part of balance, because it helps even out your weight over the skates. This keeps you from falling and helps you glide smoothly and work up some speed. Keep your head and chin up and imagine that they are connected with an imaginary line that runs down the center of your chest and connects with the toes of both of your feet.

It's also important to know how to stop. The basic stop is called a snowplow. Keeping both knees bent, shift your weight to one foot, then turn the other foot inward at an angle. Gradually shift your weight to the angled foot, which will slow you down and eventually bring you to a stop. A hockey stop is a more advanced move. To do it, quickly turn your feet sideways until they are perpendicular to the direction you were moving, putting more weight on your back foot.

Fun Facts

- The "Axel," a figure skating jump, is named for Axel Paulsen, who performed the first jump ever during a competition in 1882.
- In order to compete in the Olympics, figure skaters must be at least 15 years old.
- The blade on a figure skate is only 3-4 millimeters thick — that's the same width as two pennies.

Snow Skiing

If you think you're too young to learn how to ski, think again.

Gear Up

Skis. Are your skis the right size? If the tip of your upright ski reaches your face between your nose and chin, they are. If you're a beginner, shorter skis will be easier to control. The bindings (the part that holds your boot to the ski) are the most important parts of the ski—to make sure they don't break, get them tested regularly by a pro.

Ski boots. Make sure your boots fit and are comfortable. In general, ski boots are 1/2 size smaller than your normal shoe size.

Ski helmets. Be a trendsetter by picking up the helmet habit. Choose an American Society for Testing and Materials (ASTM) approved model that fits right, is ventilated, and doesn't affect your hearing or field of vision.

Ski poles. Ski poles are used to give you balance and help you get up if you fall, or need to side-step up a hill.

Goggles. Goggles are important to protect your eyes from flying dirt or snow, as well as stopping the sun's glare while whooshing down the slopes. Some goggles come with fun tinted lenses. If you don't have goggles, you can use sunglasses instead.

If you are renting equipment, the staff at the ski shop can help you find all the right stuff.

Stay Warm On The Slopes

- Long underwear to keep you warm and absorb sweat.
- Insulated tops and pants such as sweaters and leggings—this layer should be warm, but not baggy.
- Ski pants and jackets to protect you from snow and wetness.
- A hat, because 60 percent of heat loss is through the head.

Play It Safe

If you can, sign up for lessons from a ski school, even if you've taken lessons before—your instructor can teach you all the right moves, for beginners as well as for more advanced students.

The key to skiing is control of your equipment and your speed. If you feel yourself start to lose control, fall onto your backside or your side and don't attempt to get up until you stop sliding.

The easiest way to get hurt while skiing is to try a run or a move that is too hard. Always ski on trails that match your skill level and never attempt a jumping move, or other trick, unless taught by an instructor.

Did you know that it is just as important to drink water when you are active in the cold as in the heat? Why? Higher altitudes and colder air can cause your body to lose water. If you experience dizziness or have dry mouth, headache or muscle cramps, take a water break. A good rule would be to drink water or sports drinks before, during, and after your ski runs.

Always check the snow conditions of the slope before you go up—you'll need to ski differently in icy conditions than you would if you were on wet snow or in deep powder.

Altitude can zap your energy. Don't push it. Ski the easier runs later in the day when you are tired. Most importantly—know when to quit.

While on the slopes, set a meeting time and place to check in with your parents or friends. And always ski with a buddy. And wear plenty of sunblock, because those rays are strong on the mountain due to high altitude and reflection off the snow.

Responsibility Code for Skiers

- Always stay in control and be able to stop or avoid other people or objects.
- People ahead of you have the right of way. It is your responsibility to avoid them.
- Do not stop where you obstruct a trail or are not visible from above.
- Whenever starting downhill or merging into a trail, look uphill and yield to others.
- Always use devices to help prevent runaway equipment.
- Observe all posted signs and warnings. Keep off closed trails and out of closed areas.
- Before using any lift, you must have the knowledge and ability to load, ride, and unload safely.
- Watch out for the sun! Wear a t-shirt and sunscreen to make sure you don't get sunburned.

How To Play

Skiing can be done as a fun activity with your family or friends, and as your skills increase, you might even want to ski competitively There are several main skiing categories including alpine skiing, which is the fast-n-furious downhill skiing; freestyle skiing, in which skiers perform jumps and tricks over moguls (large bumps on the ski slope) while skiing downhill; and cross country skiing, where skiers race long distances over flatter land.

Here are some key tips to get you started:

Lift on. To get on a lift, put both your poles in your inside hand. Turn to the outside and watch for the next chair. As it gets to you, grab the outside pole and sit normally on the chair. Keep your skis apart, with the tips up, as you're lifted off the ground.

Lift off. To get off the lift, grab a pole in each hand, but don't put on your wrist straps. Point the pole tips toward the outside of the chair, and hold them up so they don't catch on the snow. Hold the bar on the outside of the chair for balance, relax your legs, and ease yourself forward, pushing off once your skis touch the snow. Don't stand up until the chair has passed over the top of the mound, and move away from the chairlift before you prepare to ski so that others can get off behind you.

Getting up after a fall. Make sure your skis are below you on the hill. Grab the top of both poles in one hand, grab the bottom of both with the other, and plant your poles in the snow just above your hip. Push up with both arms to shift yourself forward and over your skis. Make sure your weight is forward and over your skis before you stand up.

Fun Facts

- Competitive freestyle skiers can jump as high as a 3 or 4 story building, when performing tricks in the air.
- Before it was a sport, skiing was used as a form of transportation in the mountains of Europe.
- Men are allowed to compete in the Olympic ski jumping event, but women are not.

Part Five
Sports Safety

Chapter 42

Fitness Safety Tips

Being active can be great for you and great fun—but not if you get hurt. Stay smart, safe, and strong. In this chapter, you can find some general physical activity safety tips, about warming up and cooling down, avoiding injuries like knee problems, and concussions.

Physical Activity Safety Tips

Take these basic steps to stay safe:

- Be active regularly. Being active regularly builds fitness, and fit folks have a lower chance of getting hurt.

- Build up slowly. Pick activities you can do now, and then slowly challenge yourself. You might add to how often you're active or to how long you're active each time. For example, maybe add five minutes to your workout every week or two.

- Value variety. Try to do a mix of activities, so you don't put too much strain on the same parts of your body all the time.

- Be careful on hot or humid days. If possible, move your exercise indoors. That's also a good idea on days with a lot of air pollution. If you're going to be outside, rest in the shade, take breaks, and drink lots of water.

- Drink plenty of fluids. You need to drink before, during, and after activity. Read more about what to drink when working out.

About This Chapter: This chapter includes text excerpted from "Fitness—Physical Activity Safety Tips For Girls," girlshealth.gov, Office on Women's Health (OWH), March 27, 2015.

- Find safe places. Try to stay away from traffic and dark areas, for example. And avoid places with a lot of holes or other things that could make you fall.

- Follow the rules of the game. Remember that many of the rules were made just to keep you safe. Learn more about safety in sports.

- Always use the right safety equipment. Make sure that your any safety gear fits right and is in good shape.

Warming Up And Cooling Down

Warming up is a good idea. Becoming active too fast can put too much stress on your body. To get going safely, you can just do your activity at a slower pace for 10 minutes.

After you warm up, try stretching your muscles. You also can stretch at the end of your workout. Stretching combined with warming up and strengthening exercises may help prevent injuries. Check out our stretches.

What about a cool-down after being active? Cooling down may not be essential for everyone. Still, stopping suddenly may be risky for some people, and cooling down is pretty simple. If your heart rate and breathing got faster during your workout, your cool-down should slowly get them back to normal. You can do the same activity you were doing, but do it more slowly. For example, if you've been walking fast for 45 minutes, you can walk slowly instead for around 10 minutes.

Safety Equipment

From helmets to shoes, the right equipment can help keep you safe when playing sports or being active.

Helmets

Helmets help when there's a risk of falling or getting hit in the head, like in baseball, softball, biking, skiing, horseback riding, skateboarding, and inline skating. Make sure you wear a helmet that is made for the activity you are doing. And make sure you know how it is supposed to fit. In some states, the law says you have to wear a helmet while biking. Bike helmets should come with a special sticker from the U.S. Consumer Product Safety Commission (CPSC).

Special Eye Protection

Special eye protection helps prevent many sports-related eye injuries. Sports that have a high risk of eye injury include basketball, baseball, hockey, and racquet sports. Regular glasses or sunglasses will not keep your eyes safe from injury. If you wear regular glasses, the protective eyewear goes over them. If you wear goggles, they should fit snugly and have cushioning for a comfortable fit. Goggles made from a special material called polycarbonate are extremely strong. Ask your coach or eye doctor what type of eye protection you may need.

Mouth Guards

Mouth guards protect your mouth, teeth, and tongue. They offer protection in soccer, lacrosse, basketball, baseball, cheerleading, and other activities in which you could get hit in the mouth. You can get mouth guards at sport stores or from your dentist.

Pads For Your Wrists, Knees, And Elbows

Pads for your wrists, knees, and elbows can help prevent lots of injuries, including broken bones. They are important for activities such as inline skating, snowboarding, and hockey. In some sports, like soccer, your coach may require shin guards, which are pads to protect your lower leg.

Shoes

Shoes need to fit well and be right for your sport. Check with your coach or an athletic shoe salesperson about what shoes to wear. Also ask how often they need to be replaced.

Avoiding Injuries

Avoiding Knee Injuries

Knee injuries happen pretty often to young people. One of the most common knee injuries is a torn anterior cruciate ligament, called ACL for short. Teenage girls get these injuries a lot more than guys do. Why? Possibly because of the way girls' bodies are made or because of the way girls use them.

If you have a torn ACL, you might have one or all of the following symptoms:

- A "popping" sound at the time of the injury

- Pain

- Not being able to put weight on your knee

- Swelling

If you think you have any kind of injury to your knee, you should stop using it. Tell your parent or guardian right away (or, if you are at school, tell your coach or teacher). Treatment for a torn ACL may include surgery and physical therapy. Don't play again until your doctor says you can.

Your best bet is to try to prevent an ACL injury. Talk to your coach or gym teacher about what you can do. Special exercises can help build strength and flexibility, for example. You also can learn safer ways to do riskier movements, like making sure to bend your knees when you jump.

Protecting Your Bones

Your teenage years are the most important time for building strong bones. Physical activity, calcium, and vitamin D help build strong bones. Having strong bones can help prevent osteoporosis, which is a disease that can put you at risk for broken bones when you get older.

Sometimes, girls can develop osteoporosis when they're young. This doesn't happen very often. But it can happen if you get a lot of exercise from activities like competitive sports but you don't eat enough healthy food. Osteoporosis can ruin a female athlete's career because it may lead to frequent or serious injuries.

If you exercise a lot like in a competitive sport, make sure to eat a variety of healthy foods, including ones with calcium and vitamin D to protect your bones.

Not sure how much food you need? Every person is different, but generally teenage girls who are active for about an hour a day need between 2,000 and 2,400 calories every day. (For example, a 16-year-old girl who is a healthy weight and runs for an hour five days a week can eat around 2,200 calories each day.)

Do you do high-impact activities, like running or gymnastics? Vitamin D also may help lower your risk of getting tiny cracks in your bones, called stress fractures. You can do other things to help protect your bones from stress fractures, too. These include:

- Making sure to use the right equipment, like wearing running shoes for running
- Strengthening your muscles, so they can help protect your bones
- Taking a break from your high-impact activity at least one day each week
- Increasing how hard you work out only a little bit at a time
- Making sure to rest if you start to feel pain

Concussion

A concussion is a type of brain injury. It can happen when your head gets hit. But it also can happen when another part of your body gets hit in a way that the force goes all the way to your brain. Concussion is a possible risk for girls who play basketball, soccer, lacrosse, and other sports. To lower the chances of getting a concussion, always make sure to follow any rules of your sport and to use the right equipment.

Symptoms of a concussion can happen right away or several hours later. They include:

- Headache

- Not being able to remember things well

- Feeling dazed, confused, or dizzy

- Nausea or vomiting

- Blurred vision

- Being sensitive to noise or light

- Having slurred speech or saying things that don't make sense

- Not being able to concentrate

- Feeling overly tired

- Passing out (but often a person with a concussion doesn't pass out)

Girls may have different concussion symptoms than boys. In a recent study, girls were more likely to feel drowsy and sensitive to noise. Those signs can be harder to notice than boys' symptoms, which most often were confusion and not remembering things.

If you get a concussion, you must rest your body and your mind. If you think you might have a concussion, you should stop playing right away. If you have a concussion, make sure to follow all your doctor's instructions for healing, even if you start to feel better. When can you play again? When a doctor or other licensed health professional trained in concussions says you can.

Safety And Team Sports

Team sports are fun and a great way to stay fit. One sport that has been growing in popularity—but also in riskiness—is cheerleading. Whatever your sport, remember to follow all the safety rules.

What To Do If You've Had An Injury

It's very important to be careful about injuries. Make sure to:

- Stop doing the activity that you think caused the injury

- Tell your parents or guardian or your doctor if any of these happens:

- You have pain that is very bad, gets worse, or lasts more than a few days

- There is swelling where you got hurt

- The pain gets in the way of your activities or sleep

- Your injury is causing numbness

- Follow your doctor's instructions on how to care for your injury and deal with any pain

- Rest for as long as your doctor says and don't play again until your doctor gives you the okay, or you will risk not getting better

Chapter 43

Safety Tips For Runners

One of the most popular ways to improve and maintain our fitness levels is through running. While injuries can occur during all activities, running carries with a few common injuries that must be dealt with appropriately. Here are a few strategies to help someone overcome common running injuries so they can continue to strive toward their fitness goals.

1. **Create a customized exercise plan**

   If your goal is to improve your speed during the 1.5-mile run, but you are unable to run 30 minutes without stopping, you need to create a plan to increase your endurance first and then tackle your speed goals. This relatively short goal generally requires runners to create an eight to 12-week exercise plan. If your goal is to run a marathon, you are probably looking at building a plan lasting between 16 to 24 weeks or more.

2. **Be patient and manage your expectations**

   Most of us lack sufficient patience when it comes to our expectations for exercise. Most runners would be well served to adopt a mindset where patience is the first thing considered when making decisions about training, analyzing training and coping with injuries. When you get injured, you must fight the natural feeling of impatience. You're injured. It happens. The key now is to focus on addressing the injury appropriately and to put the original training plan on hold for a bit.

3. **Take advantage of physical therapy**

   You need to appropriately identify the injury and then work on rehabilitating that injury. If you continue to press on with your current exercise plan, you'll not only

About This Chapter: This chapter includes text excerpted from "Overcoming And Avoiding Running Injuries" Air Force Public Affairs Agency (AFPAA), September 5, 2014. Reviewed September 2017.

prevent adequate healing of the current injury, but you'll also run a very high risk of creating a secondary injury as your body over-stresses another muscle or joint when it tries to compensate for the original injury.

4. **Seek advice from certified health professionals**

Once you're ready to resume your training and exercise plan, seek out help from a certified health and wellness professional. You can't just jump back into your training program where you left off before being injured. The program must be adapted, and you may even have to adapt your overall fitness goals.

5. **Persevere, and adjust plans and goals accordingly**

It's imperative that you accept you had an injury, and you may have to adjust your original goal and plan and create new short and long-term goals. Your goal shouldn't be only about your "race." Your goal should be about the journey of getting to the race and achieving your goals. This requires perseverance to be flexible and adapt as injuries occur. That perseverance makes achieving your goal that much sweeter. Once you accomplish one of your goals, start again. New goal. New plan.

Running injuries may seem inevitable. However, if you deal with your running injuries appropriately, it never has to mean your running days are over.

Chapter 44

Helmets

Hard Facts About Helmets

If you like recreational activities that involve wheels, concrete or asphalt, then protect your brain by wearing a helmet. Helmets with a U.S. Consumer Product Safety Commission (CPSC) approval are good for biking and in-line skating and are available in most sporting goods stores. "Multi-sport" helmets with a Snell B-95 approval are designed for skateboarding, roller-skating, and riding scooters as well as biking and in-line skating. Snell B-95 rated helmets provide more protection but you may have to check out more stores to find one.

Your helmet should sit flat on your head—make sure it is level and is not tilted back or forward. The front of the helmet should sit low—about two finger widths above your eyebrows to protect your forehead. The straps on each side of your head should form a "Y" over your ears, with one part of the strap in front of your ear, and one behind—just below your earlobes. If the helmet leans forward, adjust the rear straps. If it tilts backward, tighten the front straps. Buckle the chinstrap securely at your throat so that the helmet feels snug on your head and does not move up and down or from side to side.

About This Chapter: Text under the heading "Hard Facts About Helmets" is excerpted from "Your Safety—Hard Facts About Helmets," Centers for Disease Control and Prevention (CDC), May 9, 2015; Text under the heading "Frequently Asked Questions About Helmet And Head Safety" is excerpted from "Sports Fitness And Recreation Bicycles—Which Helmet For Which Activity?" U.S. Consumer Product Safety Commission (CPSC), July 2014. Reviewed September 2017.

Helmets—Fact or Fiction?

Fiction: Helmets aren't cool.

Fact: Who says helmets can't be cool? If you're shopping for a helmet, there are lots of options, so you can pick out your favorite color. Or decorate your helmet with stickers and reflectors to show your personal style. Helmets are designed to help prevent injuries to your head, 'cause a serious fall or crash can cause permanent brain damage or death. And that's definitely not cool.

Fiction: Helmets just aren't comfortable.

Fact: Today's helmets are lightweight, well ventilated, and have lots of padding. Try on your helmet to make sure it fits properly and comfortably on your head before you buy it.

Fiction: Really good riders don't need to wear helmets.

Fact: Bike crashes or collisions can happen at any time. Even professional bike racers get in serious wrecks. In three out of four bike crashes, bikers usually get some sort of injury to their head.

Frequently Asked Questions About Helmet And Head Safety

Why Are Helmets So Important?

For many recreational activities, wearing a helmet can reduce the risk of a severe head injury and even save your life.

How Does A Helmet Protect My Head?

During a typical fall or collision, much of the impact energy is absorbed by the helmet, rather than your head and brain.

Does This Mean That Helmets Prevent Concussions?

No. No helmet design has been proven to prevent concussions. The materials that are used in most of today's helmets are engineered to absorb the high impact energies that can produce skull fractures and severe brain injuries. However, these materials have not been proven to counteract the energies believed to cause concussions. Beware of claims that a particular helmet can reduce or prevent concussions.

To protect against concussion injury, play smart. Learn the signs and symptoms of a concussion so that after a fall or collision, you can recognize the symptoms, get proper treatment, and prevent additional injury.

Are All Helmets The Same?

No. There are different helmets for different activities. Each type of helmet is made to protect your head from the kind of impacts that typically are associated with a particular activity or sport. Be sure to wear a helmet that is appropriate for the particular activity you're involved in. Helmets designed for other activities may not protect your head as effectively.

How Can I Tell Which Helmet Is The Right One To Use?

There are safety standards for most types of helmets. Bicycle and motorcycle helmets must comply with mandatory federal safety standards. Helmets for many other recreational activities are subject to voluntary safety standards. Helmets that meet the requirements of a mandatory or voluntary safety standard are designed and tested to protect the user from receiving a skull fracture or severe brain injury while wearing the helmet. For example, all bicycle helmets manufactured after 1999 must meet the CPSC bicycle helmet standard (16 C.F.R. part 1203); helmets meeting this standard provide protection against skull fractures and severe brain injuries when the helmet is used properly.

The protection that the appropriate helmet can provide is dependent upon achieving a proper fit and wearing it correctly; for many activities, chin straps are specified in the standard, and they are essential for the helmet to function properly. For example, the bicycle standard requires that chin straps be strong enough to keep the helmet on the head and in the proper position during a fall or collision.

Helmets that meet a particular standard will contain a special label or marking that indicates compliance with that standard (usually found on the liner inside of the helmet, on the exterior surface, or attached to the chin strap). Don't rely solely on the helmet's name or appearance, or claims made on the packaging, to determine whether the helmet meets the appropriate requirements for your activity.

Don't choose style over safety. When choosing a helmet, avoid helmets that contain non-essential elements that protrude from the helmet (e.g., horns, Mohawks)—these may look interesting, but they may prevent the helmet's smooth surface from sliding after a fall, which could lead to injury.

Don't add anything to the helmet, such as stickers, coverings, or other attachments that aren't provided with the helmet, as such items can negatively affect the helmet's performance.

Avoid novelty and toy helmets that are made only to look like the real thing; such helmets are not made to comply with any standard and can be expected to offer little or no protection.

Are There Helmets That I Can Wear For More Than One Activity?

Yes, but only a few. For example, you can wear a CPSC-compliant bicycle helmet while bicycling, recreational in-line skating or roller skating, or riding a kick scooter.

Are There Any Activities For Which One Should Not Wear A Helmet?

Yes. Children should not wear a helmet when playing on playgrounds or climbing trees. If a child wears a helmet during these activities, the helmet's chin strap can get caught on the equipment or tree branches and pose a risk of strangulation. The helmet may also prevent a child's head from moving through an opening that the body can fit through, and entrap the child by his/her head.

How Can I Tell If My Helmet Fits Properly?

A helmet should be both comfortable and snug. Be sure that the helmet is worn so that it is level on your head—not tilted back on the top of your head or pulled too low over your forehead. Once on your head, the helmet should not move in any direction, back-to-front or side-to-side. For helmets with a chin strap, be sure the chin strap is securely fastened so that the helmet doesn't move or fall off during a fall or collision. If you buy a helmet for a child, bring the child with you so that the helmet can be tested for a good fit. Carefully examine the helmet and the accompanying instructions and safety literature.

What Can I Do If I Have Trouble Fitting The Helmet?

Depending on the type of helmet, you may have to apply the foam padding that comes with the helmet, adjust the straps, adjust the air bladders, or make other adjustments specified by the manufacturer. If these adjustments do not work, consult with the store where you bought the helmet or with the helmet manufacturer. Do not add extra padding or parts, or make any adjustments that are not specifically outlined in the manufacturer's instructions. Do not wear a helmet that does not fit correctly.

Will I Need To Replace A Helmet After An Impact?

That depends on the severity of the impact and whether the helmet was designed to withstand one impact (a single-impact helmet) or more than one impact (a multiple-impact helmet). For example, bicycle helmets are designed to protect against the impact from just a single fall, such as a bicyclist's fall onto the pavement. The foam material in the helmet will crush to absorb the impact energy during a fall or collision. The materials will not protect you again from an additional impact. Even if there are no visible signs of damage to the helmet, you must replace it after such an event.

Other helmets are designed to protect against multiple impacts. Two examples are football and ice hockey helmets. These helmets are designed to withstand multiple impacts of the type associated with the respective activities. However, you may still have to replace the helmet after one severe impact if the helmet has visible signs of damage, such as a cracked shell or permanent dent in the shell or liner. Consult the manufacturer's instructions or certification stickers on the helmet for guidance on when the helmet should be replaced.

How Long Are Helmets Supposed To Last?

Follow the guidance provided by the manufacturer. In the absence of such guidance, it may be prudent to replace your helmet within 5–10 years of purchase, a decision that can be based, at least in part, on how much the helmet was used, how it was cared for, and where it was stored. Cracks in the shell or liner, a loose shell, marks on the liner, fading of the shell, evidence of crushed foam in the liner, worn straps, and missing pads or other parts, are all reasons to replace a helmet. Regular replacement may minimize any reduced effectiveness that could result from degradation of materials over time, and allow you to take advantage of recent advances in helmet protection.

Chapter 45

Clothes And Shoes For Workout Comfort And Safety

Wondering what to wear when you work out? Well, lots of activities don't require any special clothes. Sometimes, your clothes do matter.

Choosing Workout Clothes

When picking a workout outfit, remember:

- **Don't wear clothes that are very tight.** You need to be able to move freely. And if you want to stay cool, air needs to reach your skin so it can dry your sweat.

- **Color matters (really).** In the summer, lighter colors will help you keep cooler. In the winter, dark clothes trap light and help you stay warm.

- **Wear layers when it is cold out.** You can take some off as you warm up.

- **Think about your head.** Wear a hat or cap for sun protection. In cold weather, wear wool or ski caps to stay warm.

- **Find the right fabric.** If you are going to sweat, you may be more comfortable in material that soaks up wetness. Try a synthetic, like polypropylene. Cotton may be less comfortable because it stays wet longer.

- **Consider wearing a comfortable sports bra.** Wearing a supportive sports bra can help protect your breasts and keep them from bouncing painfully while exercising. Try on a few to see which style you prefer. If you need help finding the right fit, ask for help in a department store or bra store.

About This Chapter: This chapter includes text excerpted from "What To Wear To Work Out," girlshealth.gov, Office on Women's Health (OWH), March 27, 2015.

How To Pick The Right Workout Shoes

Check your shoes regularly and replace them when they're worn out. You need new shoes when:

- The tread is worn out
- Your feet feel tired after activity
- Your shins, knees, or hips hurt after activity

(Source: "Fitness Shoes And Clothes," Go4Life, National Institutes of Health (NIH).)

Wearing the right shoes when you work out is very important. To find the right pair, follow these tips:

- **Make sure your shoes protect your feet.** They should be sturdy and have cushioned soles. They should also have arch supports (the raised part inside that curves under the bottom of your foot).

- **Make sure the shoe is right for what you do.** If you plan to run or play a certain sport a lot, consider shoes made for that activity. Tennis players should wear tennis shoes and runners should wear running shoes, for example. Ask a sports shoe salesperson for help.

- **Get the right fit.** Ask a salesperson to measure your foot and then to check the fit. The wrong fit can hurt or even cause foot problems. Try to shop at the end of the day when your feet are a little larger (just like they are when you exercise). Also, when trying on shoes, wear the kind of socks you wear to work out.

Don't use any type running shoes for other sports, as they are not made for lateral movements, making ankle sprains more likely. They also last longer and maintain cushioning better if only used for running. Use only good quality court shoes or cross-trainers for other conditioning activities. Wrestling shoes are recommended for defensive tactics training on matted floors.

(Source: "Starting A Running Program," U.S. Customs and Border Protection (CBP).)

Chapter 46

Increasing Activity Safely

Although physical activity has many health benefits, injuries and other adverse events do sometimes happen. The most common injuries affect the musculoskeletal system (the bones, joints, muscles, ligaments, and tendons). Other adverse events can also occur during activity, such as overheating and dehydration. On rare occasions, people have heart attacks during activity.

The good news is that scientific evidence strongly shows that physical activity is safe for almost everyone. Moreover, the health benefits of physical activity far outweigh the risks. Still, people may hesitate to become physically active because of concern they'll get hurt. For these people, there is even more good news: They can take steps that are proven to reduce their risk of injury and adverse events. The guidelines in this chapter provide advice to help people do physical activity safely. Most advice applies to people of all ages.

Physical Activity Is Safe For Almost Everyone

Most people are not likely to be injured when doing moderate-intensity activities in amounts that meet the *Physical Activity Guidelines For Americans*. However, injuries and other adverse events do sometimes happen. The most common problems are musculoskeletal injuries. Even so, studies show that only one such injury occurs for every 1,000 hours of walking for exercise, and fewer than four injuries occur for every 1,000 hours of running.

Both physical fitness and total amount of physical activity affect risk of musculoskeletal injuries. People who are physically fit have a lower risk of injury than people who are not.

About This Chapter: This chapter includes text excerpted from "Chapter 6: Safe And Active," Office of Disease Prevention and Health Promotion (ODPHP), U.S. Department of Health and Human Services (HHS), September 6, 2017.

People who do more activity generally have a higher risk of injury than people who do less activity. So what should people do if they want to be active and safe? The best strategies are to:

- Be regularly physically active to increase physical fitness; and

- Follow the other guidance in this chapter (especially increasing physical activity gradually over time) to minimize the injury risk from doing medium to high amounts of activity.

Following these strategies may reduce overall injury risk. Active people are more likely to have an activity related injury than inactive people. But they appear less likely to have non-activity-related injuries, such as work-related injuries or injuries that occur around the home or from motor vehicle crashes.

Key Guidelines For Safe Physical Activity

To do physical activity safely and reduce risk of injuries and other adverse events, people should follow these guidelines:

- Understand the risks and yet be confident that physical activity is safe for almost every-one.

- Choose to do types of physical activity that are appropriate for their current fitness level and health goals, because some activities are safer than others.

- Increase physical activity gradually over time whenever more activity is necessary to meet guidelines or health goals. Inactive people should "start low and go slow" by gradually increasing how often and how long activities are done.

- Protect themselves by using appropriate gear and sports equipment, looking for safe environments, following rules and policies, and making sensible choices about when, where, and how to be active.

- Be under the care of a healthcare provider if they have chronic conditions or symptoms. People with chronic conditions and symptoms should consult their healthcare provider about the types and amounts of activity appropriate for them.

Choose Appropriate Types And Amounts Of Activity

People can reduce their risk of injury by choosing appropriate types of activity. The safest activities are moderate intensity and low impact, and don't involve purposeful collision or contact. Walking for exercise, gardening or yard work, bicycling or exercise cycling, dancing, swimming, and golf are activities with the lowest injury rates. In the amounts commonly done by adults, walking (a moderate-intensity and low-impact activity) has a third or less of the injury risk of running (a vigorous-intensity and higher impact activity).

The risk of injury for a type of physical activity can also differ according to the purpose of the activity. For example, recreational bicycling or bicycling for transportation leads to fewer injuries than training for and competing in bicycle races. People who have had a past injury are at risk of injuring that body part again. The risk of injury can be reduced by performing appropriate amounts of activity and setting appropriate personal goals. Performing a variety of different physical activities may also reduce the risk of overuse injury.

Increase Physical Activity Gradually Over Time

Scientific studies indicate that the risk of injury to bones, muscles, and joints is directly related to the gap between a person's usual level of activity and a new level of activity. The size of this gap is called the amount of overload. Creating a small overload and waiting for the body to adapt and recover reduces the risk of injury. When amounts of physical activity need to be increased to meet the Guidelines or personal goals, physical activity should be increased gradually over time, no matter what the person's current level of physical activity.

Scientists have not established a standard for how to gradually increase physical activity over time. The following recommendations give general guidance for inactive people and those with low levels of physical activity on how to increase physical activity:

- Use relative intensity (intensity of the activity relative to a person's fitness) to guide the level of effort for aerobic activity.

- Generally start with relatively moderate-intensity aerobic activity. Avoid relatively vigorous-intensity activity, such as shoveling snow or running. Adults with a low level of fitness may need to start with light activity, or a mix of light- to moderate-intensity activity.

- First, increase the number of minutes per session (duration), and the number of days per week (frequency) of moderate-intensity activity. Later, if desired, increase the intensity.

- Pay attention to the relative size of the increase in physical activity each week, as this is related to injury risk. For example, a 20-minute increase each week is safer for a person who does 200 minutes a week of walking (a 10 percent increase), than for a person who does 40 minutes a week (a 50 percent increase).

The available scientific evidence suggests that adding a small and comfortable amount of light- to moderate–intensity activity, such as 5 to 15 minutes of walking per session, 2 to 3 times a week, to one's usual activities has a low risk of musculoskeletal injury and no known risk of severe cardiac events. Because this range is rather wide, people should consider three factors in individualizing their rate of increase: age, level of fitness, and prior experience.

Age

The amount of time required to adapt to a new level of activity probably depends on age. Youth and young adults probably can safely increase activity by small amounts every week or 2. Older adults appear to require more time to adapt to a new level of activity, in the range of 2 to 4 weeks.

Level Of Fitness

Less fit adults are at higher risk of injury when doing a given amount of activity, compared to fitter adults. Slower rates of increase over time may reduce injury risk. This guidance applies to overweight and obese adults, as they are commonly less physically fit.

Prior Experience

People can use their experience to learn to increase physical activity over time in ways that minimize the risk of overuse injury. Generally, if an overuse injury occurred in the past with a certain rate of progression, a person should increase activity more slowly the next time.

Take Appropriate Precautions

Taking appropriate precautions means using the right gear and equipment, choosing safe environments in which to be active, following rules and policies, and making sensible choices about how, when, and where to be active.

Use Protective Gear And Appropriate Equipment

Using personal protective gear can reduce the frequency of injury. Personal protective gear is something worn by a person to protect a specific body part. Examples include helmets, eyewear and goggles, shin guards, elbow and knee pads, and mouthguards.

Using appropriate sports equipment can also reduce risk of injury. Sports equipment refers to sport or activity-specific tools, such as balls, bats, sticks, and shoes.

For the most benefit, protective equipment and gear should be the right equipment for the activity, appropriately fitted, appropriately maintained, and used consistently and correctly.

Be Active In Safe Environments

People can reduce their injury risks by paying attention to the places they choose to be active. To help themselves stay safe, people can look for:

- Physical separation from motor vehicles, such as sidewalks, walking paths, or bike lanes;

- Neighborhoods with traffic-calming measures that slow down traffic;

- Places to be active that are well-lighted, where other people are present, and that are well-maintained (no litter, broken windows);

- Shock-absorbing surfaces on playgrounds;

- Well-maintained playing fields and courts without holes or obstacles;

- Breakaway bases at baseball and softball fields; and

- Padded and anchored goals and goal posts at soccer and football fields.

Follow Rules And Policies That Promote Safety

Rules, policies, legislation, and laws are potentially the most effective and wide-reaching way to reduce activity-related injuries. To get the benefit, individuals should look for and follow these rules, policies, and laws. For example, policies that promote the use of bicycle helmets reduce the risk of head injury among cyclists. Rules against diving into shallow water at swimming pools prevent head and neck injuries.

Make Sensible Choices About How, When, And Where To Be Active

A person's choices can obviously influence the risk of adverse events. By making sensible choices, injuries and adverse events can be prevented. Consider weather conditions, such as extremes of heat and cold. For example, during very hot and humid weather, people lessen the chances of dehydration and heat stress by:

- Exercising in the cool of early morning as opposed to mid-day heat;

- Switching to indoor activities (playing basketball in the gym rather than on the playground);

- Changing the type of activity (swimming rather than playing soccer);

- Lowering the intensity of activity (walking rather than running); and

- Paying close attention to rest, shade, drinking enough fluids, and other ways to minimize effects of heat.

Exposure to air pollution is associated with several adverse health outcomes, including asthma attacks and abnormal heart rhythms. People who can modify the location or time of exercise may wish to reduce these risks by exercising away from heavy traffic and industrial sites, especially during rush hour or times when pollution is known to be high. However, current evidence indicates that the benefits of being active, even in polluted air, outweigh the risk of being inactive.

Advice From Healthcare Providers

The protective value of a medical consultation for persons with or without chronic diseases who are interested in increasing their physical activity level is not established. People without diagnosed chronic conditions (such as diabetes, heart disease, or osteoarthritis) and who do not have symptoms (such as chest pain or pressure, dizziness, or joint pain) do not need to consult a healthcare provider about physical activity.

Inactive people who gradually progress over time to relatively moderate-intensity activity have no known risk of sudden cardiac events, and very low risk of bone, muscle, or joint injuries. A person who is habitually active with moderate-intensity activity can gradually increase to vigorous intensity without needing to consult a healthcare provider. People who develop new symptoms when increasing their levels of activity should consult a healthcare provider.

Healthcare providers can provide useful personalized advice on how to reduce risk of injuries. For people who wish to seek the advice of a healthcare provider, it is particularly appropriate to do so when contemplating vigorous-intensity activity, because the risks of this activity are higher than the risks of moderate-intensity activity.

The choice of appropriate types and amounts of physical activity can be affected by chronic conditions. People with symptoms or known chronic conditions should be under the regular care of a healthcare provider. In consultation with their provider, they can develop a physical activity plan that is appropriate for them. People with chronic conditions typically find that moderate-intensity activity is safe and beneficial. However, they may need to take special precautions. For example, people with diabetes need to pay special attention to blood sugar control and proper footwear during activity.

Chapter 47

Sports-Related Concussions: What Youngsters Need To Know

Each day, hundreds of thousands of young athletes practice and compete in a wide variety of sports. Physical activity, sports participation, and play in general are great ways for children and teens to build and maintain healthy bones and muscles, lower their chances for depression and chronic diseases (such as diabetes), learn leadership and teamwork skills, and do well in school. However, research shows that when it comes to concussion, young athletes are at risk.

A concussion is a type of traumatic brain injury—or TBI—caused by a bump, blow, or jolt to the head or body that causes the head and brain to move rapidly back and forth. This sudden movement can cause the brain to bounce around or twist in the skull, creating chemical changes in the brain and sometimes stretching and damaging the brain cells.

Most children and teens with a concussion feel better within a couple of weeks. However, for some, symptoms may last for months or longer and can lead to short- and long-term problems affecting how a young person thinks, acts, learns, and feels. Parents, coaches, healthcare providers, and school professionals all play an important role in supporting young athletes so that they can thrive on the playing field, at school, and in all parts of their lives.

> You can't see a concussion. Signs and symptoms of concussion can show up right after an injury or may not appear or be noticed until hours or days after the injury. It is important to watch for changes in how children or teens act or feel, if symptoms are getting worse, or if he/she just "doesn't feel right."
>
> *(Source: "A Fact Sheet For Parents," Centers for Disease Control and Prevention (CDC).)*

About This Chapter: This chapter includes text excerpted from "Concussion At Play—Opportunities To Reshape The Culture Around Concussion," Centers for Disease Control and Prevention (CDC), July 30, 2015.

Concussion Knowledge And Awareness

On The Rise

Along with the rise in the number of educational efforts on concussion, research over the last 5 years shows that the level of awareness and knowledge about concussion among these groups has grown. For example:

- The majority of youth (ages 13–18) have heard about concussion and understand the dangers of this injury.

- Most parents view concussions as a serious injury and know that continuing to play with a concussion could cause further injury or even death.

- Many coaches are aware of general concussion symptoms and understand that an athlete does not need to lose consciousness to have a concussion.

- Healthcare providers in many areas are aware of and have access to referral networks for patients with concussion.

Gaps Still Remain

Even though knowledge and awareness of concussion is growing, research shows that there are still important gaps to be filled.

- Some parents are not familiar with state concussion laws or school or league protocols on children returning to learn and play.

- Coaches may not be able to identify subtle concussion symptoms and may not be aware of the importance of managing cognitive activities following a concussion.

- Some healthcare providers do not feel they have adequate training on concussion, and the use of evidence-based and standardized assessment tools and guidelines is limited.

- While similar research about school professionals' knowledge and awareness of concussion is not currently available, the important role that school professionals play in concussion identification and management is clear.

Concussion Attitudes And Behaviors

Too Many Young Athletes Do Not Report Concussion Symptoms

Reporting a possible concussion is the most important action young athletes can take to bring their injury to light. Reporting symptoms will facilitate an athlete being properly assessed, monitored, and treated and taking needed time to heal. Yet, research shows that too many young athletes do not take this critical first step.

In one study, researchers interviewed a group of almost 800 high school athletes during the course of a season and found that:

- Sixty-nine percent of athletes with a possible concussion played with concussion symptoms.

- Forty percent of those athletes said that their coaches were not aware that they had a possible concussion.

In a different study, 50 female and male high school athletes were asked what they would do if they thought they had a concussion:

- They most commonly answered, "I would keep playing and see how I felt" or "I would take a little break and return to play."

- None said that they would stop playing entirely if they experienced concussion symptoms.

After A Concussion, Young Athletes Are Returning To Play Too Soon

Young athletes should never return to play the same day of the injury. In addition, they should not return to play until an appropriate healthcare provider says it is okay. However, many young athletes are returning to play too soon following a concussion.

In a study of 150 young patients seen in an emergency department for concussion, many did not take time to heal fully before returning to their usual activities:

- Thirty-nine percent reported returning to play on the same day of their concussion.

- More than half (58 percent) returned to play without medical clearance.

Opportunities To Reshape The Culture Around Concussion

The Way Coaches Talk About Concussion Influences Young Athletes' Decisions To Report Concussion Symptoms

Young athletes depend on their coaches for guidance and need to feel comfortable in order to report their symptoms to their coaches, athletic trainers, teammates, and parents. In fact, young athletes' beliefs about their coaches' expectations on reporting may trump their own knowledge or intention to report a possible concussion.

The way coaches talk about concussion affects young athletes' behaviors around reporting symptoms:

- Young athletes who receive negative messages from their coaches, or who are insulted by their coaches for reporting an injury, may feel pressured to keep playing with concussion symptoms.

- On the other hand, young athletes who receive positive messages from their coach and are praised for symptom reporting are more likely to report their concussion symptoms.

ACTION STEP: Coaches should foster an environment where young athletes feel comfortable reporting a concussion. Before and during the season, coaches should talk about concussion and ask young athletes to share and discuss their concerns about reporting a concussion.

WHY THIS IS IMPORTANT: Young athletes are more likely to report concussion symptoms accurately when they receive positive messages about reporting from their coach.

Young Athletes May Feel Pressure To Hide Their Concussion Symptoms

Research shows that despite the importance of reporting their concussion symptoms, many young athletes are unaware that they have a concussion or may not report a possible concussion because they:

- Do not think a concussion is serious.

- Are worried about losing their position on the team or do not want to stop playing.

- Do not want to let their coach or teammates down.

- Are concerned about jeopardizing their future sports career or about what their coach or teammates might think of them.

ACTION STEP: Coaches should keep a list of concussion signs and symptoms and a concussion action plan on hand and visibly posted where young athletes play games and practice. Coaches should review this list frequently with their athletes.

WHY THIS IS IMPORTANT: Most young athletes understand the potentially dangerous consequences of a concussion, such as long-term disability and death. Yet young athletes may be unable to identify some symptoms, like a ringing in the ears or fatigue caused by a concussion.

Coaches also may have difficulty identifying some subtle concussion signs and symptoms, such as vision problems, sensitivity to light and noise, and problems with sleep.

Young Athletes Are More Likely To Play With A Concussion During A Big Game

Young athletes may be more reluctant to tell a coach or athletic trainer about a possible concussion in a championship game compared to a regular game. Researchers presented the following situation to 58 young athletes: "During a championship game, you develop an injury that does not significantly hinder your ability to play, but could result in severe or permanent injury if you continue to play. Do you tell your coach or athletic trainer, or do you say nothing and continue to play?"

- Fifty-two percent of young athletes said they would always report an injury during a championship game or event.

- Thirty-six percent of young athletes said that they would sometimes tell their coach or athletic trainer, while 7 percent said they would never tell their coach or athletic trainer about the injury.

Similarly, the same researchers asked a group of 314 coaches if they would remove a young athlete from play with concussion symptoms in different scenarios:

- Ninety-two percent of coaches reported they would remove the young athlete from play when the importance of the game or event was not included in the scenario.

- When the scenario included a championship game, 17–20 percent of coaches indicated that they would allow a concussed athlete to keep playing.

ACTION STEP: Parents and coaches need to communicate to athletes that a concussion should be reported no matter how important the game or event seems. Athletes should know that health and safety always come first.

WHY THIS IS IMPORTANT: Parents and coaches greatly influence how athletes think about sports, such as their motivation to play, enjoyment of the sport, goals, and decision-making. Young athletes may not report their symptoms because they feel pressure from or worry about letting down their coach, parent(s), or teammates.

Healthcare Providers And School Professionals Can Help Young Athletes Successfully Return To Learn And Play

As many as a third of young athletes do not receive clear discharge instructions after going to an emergency department with concussion symptoms. When discharge instructions are provided, healthcare providers often give instructions on return to play but not on return to learn.

There is limited research about school professionals' knowledge of concussion, yet the most important action that school professionals can take is to support young athletes during their recovery process as they return to learn. A student's quality of care is improved when school professionals across the school setting work in collaboration to achieve positive school outcomes. Healthcare providers and school professionals can guide young athletes and their parents as they return to activity in the classroom and on the playing field.

ACTION STEP: Parents should receive written instructions from healthcare providers on return to learn and return to play strategies. This information needs to be given to an athlete's coach and school.

WHY THIS IS IMPORTANT: Youth athletes and their parents need guidance to support them as they return to learn and play. Coaches and school professionals will benefit from these written instructions as well. Young athletes also need to take time to heal before returning to school since thinking and learning can be difficult when the brain is still healing. In one study, 30 percent of students reported a decline in school performance or attendance after a concussion.

Creating A Safe Sport Culture

Athletes thrive when they:

- Have fun playing their sport.

- Receive positive messages and praise from their coaches for concussion symptom reporting.

- Have parents who talk with them about concussion and model and expect safe play.

- Feel comfortable reporting symptoms of a possible concussion to coaches.

- Support their teammates sitting out of play if they have concussion.

- Get written instructions from a healthcare provider on when to return to school and play.

Education Efforts Help Play A Role In Concussion Safety

Participation in concussion education may support increased symptom reporting by athletes. A survey of almost 170 high school athletes in six sports found that young athletes who were more knowledgeable about concussion were more likely to report a concussion during practice.

Another study of high school athletes who received concussion education from any source were more likely to report concussion symptoms to a coach or athletic trainer compared to athletes with no education. Specifically:

- Seventy-two percent of athletes who had received concussion education indicated that they would always notify their coach of concussion symptoms.

- Only 12 percent of athletes who had no history of concussion education stated they would always report their concussion symptoms to their coach.

Similarly, coaches who receive coaching education are more likely to correctly recognize concussion signs and symptoms and feel comfortable deciding whether an athlete needs to be evaluated for a possible concussion.

ACTION STEP: Educate young athletes and coaches on the importance of concussion throughout the season using materials that have been evaluated and shown to be effective. Education efforts should be coupled with programmatic and league policy activities.

WHY THIS IS IMPORTANT: Educational efforts should be tailored to meet the needs of and address the main concerns reported by athletes. Improving coaches' and young athletes' knowledge alone may not always result in increased concussion reporting by athletes. A pilot study implemented in 40 high schools that included standardized protocols for schools and medical providers, education and training, and coordination among the key stakeholders led to an increase in the number of concussions identified, reported, and treated.

Young Athletes Look To Parents And Coaches To Understand The Culture Of Safety

A young athlete's views and actions on the sports field are influenced by those of their parents, coaches, teammates, and even spectators. Together, these groups shape a "sports culture."

Action Steps: Expect Safe Play. Model Safe Play. Reinforce Safe Play.

Expect Safe Play

Why this is important: While not risk-free, sports are a great way for children and teens to stay healthy and can help them do well in school. Young athletes look to their coaches and parents to learn which actions are okay in the "team's culture" and how to follow safe play and the rules of the sport.

Model Safe Play

Why this is important: Children and teens learn from what they see their parents doing. In a study of parents and their children who ski and snowboard:

- Ninety-six percent of children who wore a helmet said that their parents also wore a ski or snowboard helmet.

- Among parents who did not wear a helmet, only 17 percent of their children wore one.

Reinforce Safe Play

Why this is important: As many as 25 percent of the concussions reported among high school athletes result from aggressive or illegal play activity. A culture that supports aggressive or unsportsmanlike behavior among young athletes can increase their chances of getting a concussion or other serious injury. Such an atmosphere also encourages athletes to hide concussion symptoms and keep playing when they are hurt.

Chapter 48

Tips For Exercising Safely In Adverse Weather

Exercising In Hot Weather

Understanding warm and/or hot weather definitions is very important for an athlete or just an exerciser for fitness so that they may better comprehend heat illness, preventative measures, and treatment options if necessary. Of the many relevant heat related definitions, the heat index is one of the most important.

Steadman or Heat Index: The combination of air temperature and humidity that gives a description of how the temperature feels. This is not the actual air temperature. When the heat index is at or over 90 degrees Fahrenheit, extreme caution should be considered before exercising outdoors.

Heat Illness: What Is It And How Do You Manage It?

Some recommendations on how to prevent exertional heat related illness include:

- When exercising in high heat and humidity, rest 10 minutes for every hour and change wet clothing frequently.

About This Chapter: Text beginning with the heading "Exercising In Hot Weather" is excerpted from "Fit For Duty Fit For Life—Exercising In Hot Weather," U.S. Public Health Service Commissioned Corps (PHSCC), U.S. Department of Health and Human Services (HHS), August 5, 2007. Reviewed September 2017; Text beginning with the heading "Cold Weather Safety" is © 2018 Omnigraphics. Reviewed September 2017; Text beginning with the heading "Air Pollution And Exercise—Outdoor Activity And Air Pollution" is excerpted from "Physical Activity And Air Pollution Exposure," U.S. Environmental Protection Agency (EPA), February 10, 2014. Reviewed September 2017.

- Avoid the midday sun by exercising before 10 a.m. or after 6 p.m., if possible.

- Use a sunscreen with a rating of SPF-15 or lower dependent upon skin type. Ratings above SPF-15 can interfere with the skin's thermal regulation.

- Wear light-weight and breathable clothing.

- Weigh yourself pre and post exercise. If there is a less than a 2 percent weight loss after exercise, you are considered mildly dehydrated. With a 2 percent and greater weight loss, you are considered dehydrated.

During hot weather training, dehydration occurs more frequently and has more severe consequences. Drink early and at regular intervals according to the American College of Sports Medicine (ACSM). The perception of thirst is a poor index of the magnitude of fluid deficit. Monitoring your weight loss and ingesting chilled volumes of fluid during exercise at a rate equal to that lost from sweating is a better method to preventing dehydration.

- Rapid fluid replacement is not recommended for rehydration. Rapid replacement of fluid stimulates increased urine production, which reduces the body water retention.

- Individuals involved in a short bout of exercise are generally fine with water fluid replacement of an extra 8–16 ounces. A sports drink (with salt and potassium) is suggested for exercise lasting longer than an hour, such as a marathon, and at a rate of about 16 to 24 ounces an hour depending upon the amount you sweat and the heat index.

- Replace fluids after long bouts of exercise (greater than an hour) at a rate of 16 ounces of fluid per pound of body weight lost during exercise.

- Avoid caffeinated, protein, and alcoholic drinks, e.g., colored soda, coffee, tea.

- Acclimate to exercising outdoors, altitude, and physical condition. General rule of thumb is 10–14 days for adults and 14–21 days for children (prepubescent) and older adults (> 60 years). Children and older adults are less heat tolerant and have a less effective thermoregulatory system.

- Educate and prepare yourself for outdoor activities. Many websites offer heat index calculations for your local weather conditions.

Summer weather does not have to sideline your outdoor exercise regimen. The above suggestions can help you plan and find ways to modify your routine to exercise safely in warm, hot, and humid weather.

You should take extra care when exercising in warm weather. The following tips will keep you safe in the heat:

- Exercise in the early morning or after the sun sets.
- Take frequent rest and water breaks.
- Drink water before you feel thirsty. By the time you feel thirsty, you are already dehydrated. This is especially true as you get older.
- Drink fluids before, during, and after exercise.
- Choose water or a low-calorie sport drink.
- Avoid beverages with alcohol and caffeine because these can cause dehydration.
- Wear light, loose-fitting clothing made of breathable fabric in light colors. Choose shady areas when possible.
- Reduce speed or distance as needed.
- Exercise indoors during ozone alerts, extreme heat, and very high humidity.
- Use sunscreen, hats, and sunglasses.

(Source: "Warm Weather Exercise Guidelines," U.S. Department of Veterans Affairs (VA).)

How Can You Prevent Exertional Heat Related Illnesses?

Some recommendations on how to prevent exertional heat related illness include:

- When exercising in high heat and humidity, rest 10 minutes for every hour and change wet clothing frequently.

- Avoid the midday sun by exercising before 10 a.m. or after 6 p.m., if possible.

- Use a sunscreen with a rating of SPF-15 or lower dependent upon skin type. Ratings above SPF-15 can interfere with the skin's thermal regulation.

- Wear light-weight and breathable clothing.

- Weigh yourself pre and post exercise. If there is a less than a 2 percent weight loss after exercise, you are considered mildly dehydrated. With a 2 percent and greater weight loss, you are considered dehydrated.

During hot weather training, dehydration occurs more frequently and has more severe consequences. Drink early and at regular intervals according to the American College of Sports

Medicine (ACSM). The perception of thirst is a poor index of the magnitude of fluid deficit. Monitoring your weight loss and ingesting chilled volumes of fluid during exercise at a rate equal to that lost from sweating is a better method to preventing dehydration.

- Rapid fluid replacement is not recommended for rehydration. Rapid replacement of fluid stimulates increased urine production, which reduces the body water retention.

- Individuals involved in a short bout of exercise are generally fine with water fluid replacement of an extra 8–16 ounces. A sports drink (with salt and potassium) is suggested for exercise lasting longer than an hour, such as a marathon, and at a rate of about 16 to 24 ounces an hour depending upon the amount you sweat and the heat index.

- Replace fluids after long bouts of exercise (greater than an hour) at a rate of 16 ounces of fluid per pound of body weight lost during exercise.

- Avoid caffeinated, protein, and alcoholic drinks, e.g., colored soda, coffee, tea.

- Acclimate to exercising outdoors, altitude, and physical condition. General rule of thumb is 10–14 days for adults and 14–21 days for children (prepubescent) and older adults (> 60 years). Children and older adults are less heat tolerant and have a less effective thermoregulatory system.

- Educate and prepare yourself for outdoor activities. Many websites offer heat index calculations for your local weather conditions.

Summer weather does not have to sideline your outdoor exercise regimen. The above suggestions can help you plan and find ways to modify your routine to exercise safely in warm, hot, and humid weather.

Cold Weather Safety

Winter activities like alpine skiing, snowboarding, cross-country skiing, snowshoeing, sledding, and ice skating are enjoyed by millions of people each year. Yet exercising outdoors in cold weather involves certain health risks, including potentially serious conditions like frostbite and hypothermia. Understanding the potential hazards and taking appropriate precautions allows people to stay safe and healthy while participating in winter sports.

Health Risks Of Cold-Weather Activities

Although cold-weather activities can be safe and enjoyable for most people, those with health conditions like asthma, circulatory problems, or heart disease should get approval from a doctor before starting a winter exercise program. In addition, everyone should take simple precautions like leaving information about their intended exercise route and return time with a friend or family member in case a problem should arise. Some of the common health risks associated with cold-weather activities include frostbite, hypothermia, dehydration, and slip-and-fall injuries.

Frostbite

Frostbite occurs when skin and body tissue freezes through exposure to extreme cold. Frostbite is a serious injury, as damaged tissue typically cannot regenerate and must be surgically removed. Frostbite usually affects bare skin on the face—such as the nose, cheeks, or ears—or the extremities furthest from the heart—such as the fingers and toes. In the early stages of frostbite, common symptoms include tingling, aching, burning, or stinging sensations in the affected area, followed by a loss of sensation or numbness. The skin may also appear bright red or mottled grey, and the body part may become swollen. If these signs of frostbite appear, it is important to seek shelter immediately, warm the area slowly, and seek medical treatment if feelings of numbness continue.

Hypothermia

Hypothermia occurs when the core temperature decreases to the point where the body is unable to maintain normal functions. Shivering is usually the first sign of a decrease in core temperature, as the body initiates involuntary muscle movement in an effort to generate heat. If the core temperature continues to fall, the body directs blood flow away from the extremities to protect the vital organs. At this point, motor functions begin to slow down and muscles may become rigid, causing problems with dexterity and coordination. As hypothermia reaches a severe stage, brain function is affected as well, producing such symptoms as slurred speech, confusion, irritability, and fatigue. Hypothermia becomes life-threatening if the core temperature drops from its normal 98.6°F (37°C) to around 92°F (33°C). Although hypothermia is most common in temperatures below freezing, it can occur even in 50°F (10°C) weather. Children and elderly people are more vulnerable to hypothermia than healthy adults. Other factors that increase the risk of hypothermia include inappropriate attire, wet clothing, and dehydration.

Dehydration

Although most people only worry about dehydration in hot weather, it is a serious health concern in cold weather as well. Breathing cold, dry winter air and perspiring through exercise leads to fluid loss through evaporation. In addition, the body's tendency to concentrate blood flow in the core when exposed to cold temperatures causes the kidneys to produce more urine than usual. Since these factors can increase the risk of dehydration, it is important to consume extra fluids before, during, and after winter workouts. Covering the nose and mouth with a scarf can also help reduce fluid loss.

Slips And Falls

Many cold-weather injuries occur due to issues related to poor visibility or unsafe terrain. Shortened daylight hours during the winter months forces many people to exercise at night, when temperatures are colder and they are less able to see obstacles like potholes or patches of ice. Falling and blowing snow can also limit visibility. Meanwhile, icy or snow-covered streets, sidewalks, and jogging paths can create slippery surfaces that may cause people to fall down or twist an ankle. In extreme conditions, the safest approach may be to stick to areas that are familiar and are regularly cleared of snow, or to work out indoors at a gym.

Staying Safe Outdoors In Winter

With proper precautions, outdoor exercise can be safe and enjoyable even at the peak of winter. Key features of preparing for cold-weather fitness activities include paying attention to the forecast, dressing in layers of clothing to preserve body heat, protecting the extremities from frostbite, and wearing proper safety equipment.

Check The Forecast

The first step in planning for outdoor activities in winter is being aware of the weather forecast. Snow, ice, and wind can develop quickly and create dangerous conditions for people who are unprepared. The outdoor air temperature is an important consideration, since the risk of frostbite is very low when the thermometer reads 5° Fahrenheit (-15° Celsius) or higher. In temperatures of -18°F (-28°C) or lower, however, frostbite can affect exposed skin within minutes. Exposure to moisture from rain, snow, or sweat also increases the risk of hypothermia by making it more difficult for the body to maintain its core temperature.

Watch The Wind Chill

Wind is another important thing to consider when preparing for outdoor exercise. The U.S. National Weather Service (NWS) has established the wind-chill factor as a tool to inform people about the added cooling effect of wind velocity. High wind speeds multiply the impact of cold temperatures on exposed skin, increasing the risk of frostbite and hypothermia.

Exercisers who move at high speeds, like bicyclists or alpine skiers, must also consider the effect of their own velocity on cold exposure. Riding at 15 miles per hour into a 10 mph head-wind, for instance, creates a wind-chill equivalent of 25 mph.

Dress In Layers

The key to preventing hypothermia is conserving body heat by wearing appropriate clothing. Studies have shown that wearing several layers of lightweight clothing provides better insulation than wearing a single layer of heavy clothing, because the air trapped between the layers provides a barrier to heat loss. An ideal system of cold-weather exercise clothing includes a lightweight, quick-drying synthetic fabric next to the skin, an insulating layer of fleece or wool in the middle, and a waterproof, breathable outer layer with a zipper for easy removal. It is best to avoid wearing cotton or other natural fibers that retain moisture, because wet clothing loses most of its insulating properties. It is also important to avoid overdressing because the body naturally generates heat during exercise. Since up to 40 percent of body heat escapes through the head, wearing a hat is another great way to protect against hypothermia.

Protect The Extremities

The hands, feet, and face are particularly vulnerable to frostbite because the body diverts blood flow away from the extremities to protect the core in response to cold. Layering works well for protecting the hands and feet from the effects of cold while exercising. A thin pair of synthetic socks worn under thermal socks, or thin glove liners worn beneath a heavier pair of wool or fleece-lined mittens, provides insulation as well as options for removal if one layer becomes wet or sweaty. Chemical heat packs or battery-powered socks and gloves are also available to help keep hands and feet warm in extreme temperatures. It is also important to cover the face and ears with a scarf, ski mask, headband, or balaclava.

Wear Safety Gear

To stay safe while exercising outdoors in the winter, it is important to choose the right equipment. Walking, running, or biking in low-light or snowy conditions, for instance, is significantly safer for people who wear reflective clothing and use a head lamp. Boots or shoes should provide sufficient traction on snowy or icy terrain. Experts also suggest wearing a protective helmet while participating in high-speed winter sports like alpine skiing or snowboarding. Finally, exercising in the snow amplifies the risk of sun damage to the skin and eyes, so it is important to wear sunscreen, lip balm, and sunglasses or goggles that feature protection from ultraviolet radiation.

References

1. Gestl, Jon. "Winter Weather Workouts," Topend Sports, 2004.

2. Niemann, Andrew, and Susan Yeargin. "Cold Weather Sports: Recognizing And Preventing Dehydration, Hypothermia, And Frostbite," MomsTeam, 2017.

3. "Winter Fitness: Safety Tips For Exercising Outdoors," Mayo Clinic, 2017.

Air Pollution And Exercise—Outdoor Activity And Air Pollution

- Exposure to air pollution is associated with several adverse health outcomes, including asthma attacks and abnormal heart rhythms.

- People who can modify the location or time of exercise may wish to reduce these risks by exercising away from heavy traffic and industrial sites, especially during rush hour or times when pollution is known to be high.

- However, current evidence indicates that the benefits of being active, even in polluted air, outweigh the risk of being inactive.

Air Pollution Exposure While Being Active

How Physical Activity Affects Air Pollution Dose?

- Concentration varies across microenvironments
  - When and where activity occurs
- Time spent in microenvironment
  - Duration of activity (e.g., active travel vs. driving)
- Ventilation rate correlates with intensity of activity
  - Increased ventilation rate: more breaths/minute
  - Increased velocity of breaths: forces air deeper into lungs and increases deposition fraction
  - More mouth breathing: bypasses nasal filtration
- Dose is dependent on age, sex, and body size

Air Pollution And Physical Activity Joint Health Effects

- Mortality risks vs. benefits

  - Studies on increasing active travel consistently show that benefits (physical activity) > risks (air pollution and injury)

  - Modeled predictions of hypothetical scenarios using relative risk data from literature

- Built environment plays an important role in determining air pollution and physical activity levels

Short-Term Exposure And Lung Function

- 60 adults with asthma walk for 2 hours along two different routes

- Larger decline in lung function after walking more polluted route

Long-Term Exposure And Asthma Incidence

- Playing ≥3 sports increased risk of asthma in high ozone communities, but not in low ozone communities

Chapter 49

Foods And Drinks For Physical Activity

If you're active, you need fuel. But how much do you need, and when? Keep reading to learn more.

Foods For Working Out

Everybody needs to eat a variety of healthy foods. But you may need to eat more if you are very active, like if you run several days each week or are on a sports team. That's because you need food to grow and to fuel all your activity. If you are very active but don't eat enough healthy food, your body may slow down and not work as well.

Confused about how much you need to eat? You can use the SuperTracker tool (www.supertracker.usda.gov) to find out what to eat and how much based on things like your activity level. (If you create a profile, you can get even more personalized info.) You can look at the tracker with a parent or guardian. In addition, you can get nutrition help from people like a doctor, school nurse, and nutritionist or dietitian. A coach or trainer also might be able to help.

Wondering when to eat? Try not to eat a meal right before exercising, or you could get a stomach ache. It can take a few hours to digest a big meal. After a smaller meal, waiting around an hour should be fine. If you have several athletic events in one day (such as a few tennis matches), you can eat small snacks between events.

About This Chapter: This chapter includes text excerpted from "Foods And Drinks For Physical Activity," girlshealth.gov, Office on Women's Health (OWH), March 27, 2015.

What To Drink During Physical Activity

If you are active, you need to make sure to get enough water and other fluids. Getting too little fluids can mess up your memory, concentration, athletic ability, and more. Check out some helpful tips below.

Water works! It does a great job of replacing fluids you lose when you sweat, for example. How much do you need? That depends on lots of things, including how active you are and how hot it is.

Experts suggest drinking about a cup of water an hour or two before getting active. During your activity, try to drink around a cup every 15 or 20 minutes. Keep drinking water after the activity ends and sipping throughout the day.

You may need to drink even more if you are going to be working out very hard, such as in something like competitive soccer or cross-country running. You can ask your doctor, coach, or trainer for more information.

One way to tell if you're getting enough water is to check your urine (pee). It should be light yellow. If it's dark yellow, you probably need more water.

Don't wait until you feel thirsty. If you feel thirsty, you could be getting dehydrated. Being dehydrated means that your body does not have as much fluid as it should. It can be dangerous. Signs of dehydration include:

- A dry or sticky mouth
- Having less or darker urine
- Fast heart rate
- Feeling irritable or confused
- Feeling dizzy or weak
- Having a headache

If you have any of the symptoms above, tell an adult.

What About Sports Drinks, Energy Drinks, And Vitamin Waters?

Usually, water is all you need when you are active.

Sports drinks can help athletes when they are active for more than an hour doing an intense activity, such as running, biking, or playing basketball or soccer. That's because sports drinks (such as Gatorade) have sugars and salts you lose when you work out. If you don't exercise that much, it's best to avoid sports drinks because they have extra sugar and calories that may lead to cavities and weight gain.

Energy drinks are a bad idea for teens. For one, energy drinks often have a lot of caffeine. In fact, one energy drink could have as much caffeine as 14 cans of soda. What's wrong with caffeine? It can cause problems like increased blood pressure, trouble sleeping, and feeling nervous. It's also possible caffeine may block your body's use of calcium (which you need for strong bones). Plus, energy drinks can have things that are not good for your health, like lots of added sugar.

Vitamin waters or enhanced waters have extra vitamins and minerals. They may also be packed with extra calories, artificial sweeteners, caffeine, or ingredients that may not be safe for kids. The best way for you to get the nutrients you need is by eating a wide variety of healthy foods.

What About Energy Bars?

Energy bars can give you energy. But they can also give you hundreds of extra calories. (One bar can have as many calories as a small order of fries!) That may be fine for teens who often do things that burn a lot of calories, like going on long runs or playing on the soccer team. For some teens, though, energy bars may pack on too many pounds. Instead, try other on-the-go snacks, like air-popped popcorn, whole-grain cereal, a banana, low-fat cheese sticks, or unsalted nuts.

Part Six
Overcoming Obstacles To Fitness

Chapter 50

Maintaining Fitness Motivation

Staying Motivated To Stay Active

Physical activity is a great way for people to gain substantial health benefits and maintain independence. To make physical activity a routine habit, choose activities and exercises that are fun, motivate you, and keep you interested. Keep it going. If you can stick with an exercise routine or physical activity for at least 6 months, it's a good sign that you're on your way to making physical activity a regular habit. Choose activities:

- You enjoy and believe you'll benefit from

- You can fit into your schedule

- You can do safely and correctly

- That are affordable

- That include friends or family

Keep it positive. Set realistic goals, regularly check your progress, and celebrate your accomplishments. These will help keep you on track.

About This Chapter: Text under the heading "Staying Motivated To Stay Active" is excerpted from "Staying Motivated To Stay Active," *Go4Life*, National Institutes of Health (NIH), January 23, 2009. Reviewed September 2017; Text under the heading "Make A Plan" is excerpted from "Make A Plan," *Go4Life*, National Institutes of Health (NIH), January 7, 2012. Reviewed September 2017; Text beginning with the heading "Talking With Your Healthcare Provider" is excerpted from "Stay Safe," *Go4Life*, National Institutes of Health (NIH), November 2, 2011. Reviewed September 2017; Text under the heading "Track Your Activities" is excerpted from "Track Your Activities," *Go4Life*, National Institutes of Health (NIH), December 18, 2011. Reviewed September 2017; Text under the heading "Set Your Goals" is excerpted from "Set Your Goals," *Go4Life*, National Institutes of Health (NIH), September 16, 2014. Reviewed September 2017.

Keep your eye on the prize. Focus on the benefits of regular exercise and physical activity:

- Greater ease doing daily tasks

- More energy to do the things you enjoy most

- Improved health

- Better outlook on life

Keep track of your progress.

- Track your physical activity

- Find new ways to increase your physical activity

- Update your exercise plan as you progress

The ten most common reasons people cite for not adopting more physically active lifestyles are:

- Do not have enough time to exercise

- Find it inconvenient to exercise

- Lack self-motivation

- Do not find exercise enjoyable

- Find exercise boring

- Lack confidence in their ability to be physically active (low self-efficacy)

- Fear being injured or have been injured recently

- Lack self-management skills, such as the ability to set personal goals, monitor progress, or reward progress toward such goals

- Lack encouragement, support, or companionship from family and friends, and

- Do not have parks, sidewalks, bicycle trails, or safe and pleasant walking paths convenient to their homes or offices.

(Sources: "Physical Activity—Overcoming Barriers To Physical Activity," Centers for Disease Control and Prevention (CDC).)

Make A Plan

Some people find that writing an exercise and physical activity plan helps them keep their promise to be active. See if this works for you. Be sure the plan is realistic for you to do. You might even make a contract with a friend or family member to carry out your plan. Involving another person can help you keep your commitment. Start out with realistic activities based on how physically active you are now.

Aim for moderate-intensity endurance activities on most or all days of the week. Try to do strength exercises for all of your major muscle groups on 2 or more days a week, but don't exercise the same muscle group 2 days in a row. For example, do upper-body strength exercises on Monday, Wednesday, and Friday and lower-body strength exercises on Tuesday, Thursday, and Saturday. Or, you can do strength exercises of all of your muscle groups every other day. Don't forget to include balance and flexibility exercises. You may find it helpful to keep a record of your endurance, strength, balance, and flexibility exercises. When it comes to motivation, the first few months are crucial. If you can stick with physical activities you enjoy, it's a good sign that you will be able to make exercise and physical activity a regular part of your everyday life.

Stay Safe

Almost anyone, at any age, can safely do some kind of exercise and physical activity. You can be active even if you have a long-term condition, like heart disease, diabetes, or arthritis. Staying safe while you exercise is always important, whether you're just starting a new activity or you haven't been active for a long time. Be sure to review the specific safety tips related to endurance, strength, balance, and flexibility exercises.

Talking With Your Healthcare Provider

Most people don't need to check with their healthcare provider first before doing physical activity. However, you may want to talk with your healthcare provider if you aren't used to energetic activity and you want to start a vigorous exercise program or significantly increase your physical activity. Your activity level is an important topic to discuss with your healthcare provider as part of your ongoing healthcare.

Ask how physical activity can help you, whether you should avoid certain activities, and how to modify exercises to fit your situation.

Other reasons to talk with your healthcare provider:

- Any new symptoms you haven't yet discussed

- Dizziness, shortness of breath

- Chest pain or pressure

- The feeling that your heart is skipping, racing, or fluttering

- Blood clots

- An infection or fever with muscle aches

- Unplanned weight loss

- Foot or ankle sores that won't heal

- Joint swelling

- A bleeding or detached retina, eye surgery, or laser treatment

- A hernia

- Recent hip or back surgery

Track Your Activities

Once you've put your physical activity plan into action, it's a good idea to keep track of what you're doing. Tracking your activities will help you stick with your plan and is a good way to make sure you're including all four types of exercise (endurance, strength, balance, and flexibility) on a regular basis. A record of your activities also is a great way to see your progress over time and can motivate you to keep going.

Set Your Goals

Many people find that having a firm goal in mind motivates them to move ahead on a project. Goals are most useful when they are specific, realistic, and important to you. Be sure to review your goals regularly. Using the interactive My Goals tool to help you set both short- and long-term goals and keep track of your progress. Short-term goals will help you make physical activity a regular part of your daily life. For these goals, think about the things you need to get or do to be physically active. For example, you may need to buy appropriate fitness clothes or walking shoes. Make sure your short-term goals will really help you be more active.

If you're already active, think of short-term goals to increase your level of physical activity. For example, over the next week or two, increase the amount of weight you lift or try a different kind of physical activity. No matter what your starting point, reaching your short-term goals will give you confidence to progress toward your long-term goals.

After you decide on your short-term goals, go on to identify your long-term goals. Focus on where you want to be in 6 months, a year, or 2 years from now. Long-term goals also should be realistic, personal, and important to you.

Chapter 51

You Can Be Active At Any Size

Physical activity may seem hard if you're overweight. You may get short of breath or tired quickly. Finding or affording the right clothes and equipment may be frustrating. Or, perhaps you may not feel comfortable working out in front of others.

The good news is you can overcome these challenges. Not only can you be active at any size, you can have fun and feel good at the same time.

Can Anyone Be Active?

Research strongly shows that physical activity is safe for almost everyone. The health benefits of physical activity far outweigh the risks.

The activities discussed here are safe for most people. If you have problems moving or staying steady on your feet, or if you get out of breath easily, talk with a healthcare professional before you start. You also should talk with a healthcare professional if you are unsure of your health, have any concerns that physical activity may be unsafe for you, or have:

- a chronic disease such as diabetes, high blood pressure, or heart disease

- a bone or joint problem—for example, in your back, knee, or hip—that could get worse if you change your physical activity level

About This Chapter: This chapter includes text excerpted from "Weight Management—Staying Active At Any Size," National Institute of Diabetes and Digestive and Kidney Diseases (NIDDK), July 2016.

Why Should I Be Active?

Being active may help you live longer and protect you from developing serious health problems, such as type 2 diabetes, heart disease, stroke, and certain types of cancer. Regular physical activity is linked to many health benefits, such as:

- lower blood pressure and blood glucose, or blood sugar

- healthy bones, muscles, and joints

- a strong heart and lungs

- better sleep at night and improved mood

The *Physical Activity Guidelines for Americans* define regular physical activity as at least 2½ hours a week of moderate-intensity activity, such as brisk walking. Brisk walking is a pace of 3 miles per hour or faster. A moderate-intensity activity makes you breathe harder but does not overwork or overheat you.

You may reach this goal by starting with 10 minutes of activity 3 days per week, and working up to 30 minutes a day 5 days a week. If you do even more activity, you may gain even more health benefits.

When combined with healthy eating, regular physical activity may also help you control your weight. However, research shows that even if you can't lose weight or maintain your weight loss, you still can enjoy important health benefits from regular physical activity.

Physical activity also can be a lot of fun if you do activities you enjoy and are active with other people. Being active with others may give you a chance to meet new people or spend more time with family and friends. You also may inspire and motivate one another to get and stay active.

What Do I Need To Know About Becoming Active?

Choosing physical activities that match your fitness level and health goals can help you stay motivated and keep you from getting hurt. You may feel some minor discomfort or muscle soreness when you first become active. These feelings should go away as you get used to your activity. However, if you feel sick to your stomach or have pain, you may have done too much. Go easier and then slowly build up your activity level. Some activities, such as walking or water workouts, are less likely to cause injuries.

If you have been inactive, start slowly and see how you feel. Gradually increase how long and how often you are active. If you need guidance, check with a healthcare or certified fitness professional.

Here are some tips for staying safe during physical activity:

- Wear the proper safety gear, such as a bike helmet if you are bicycling.

- Make sure any sports equipment you use works and fits properly.

- Look for safe places to be active. For instance, walk in well-lit areas where other people are around. Be active with a friend or group.

- Stay hydrated to replace the body fluids you lose through sweating and to prevent you from getting overheated.

- If you are active outdoors, protect yourself from the sun with sunscreen and a hat or protective visor and clothing.

- Wear enough clothing to keep warm in cold or windy weather. Layers are best.

If you don't feel right, stop your activity. If you have any of the following warning signs, stop and seek help right away:

- pain, tightness, or pressure in your chest or neck, shoulder, or arm

- extreme shortness of breath

- dizziness or sickness

Check with a healthcare professional about what to do if you have any of these warning signs. If your activity is causing pain in your joints, feet, ankles, or legs, you also should consult a healthcare professional to see if you may need to change the type or amount of activity you are doing.

What Kinds Of Activities Can I Do?

You don't need to be an athlete or have special skills or equipment to make physical activity part of your life. Many types of activities you do every day, such as walking your dog or going up and down steps at home or at work, may help improve your health.

Try different activities you enjoy. If you like an activity, you're more likely to stick with it. Anything that gets you moving around, even for a few minutes at a time, is a healthy start to getting fit.

Walking

Walking is free and easy to do—and you can do it almost anywhere. Walking will help you:

- burn calories

- improve your fitness

- lift your mood

- strengthen your bones and muscles

If you are concerned about safety, try walking in a shopping mall or park where it is well lit and other people are around. Many malls and parks have benches where you can take a quick break. Walking with a friend or family member is safer than walking alone and may provide the social support you need to meet your activity goals.

If you don't have time for a long walk, take several short walks instead. For example, instead of a 30-minute walk, add three 10-minute walks to your day. Shorter spurts of activity are easier to fit into a busy schedule.

Walking Tips

- Wear comfortable, well-fitting walking shoes with a lot of support, and socks that absorb sweat.

- Dress for the weather if you are walking outdoors. In cold weather, wear layers of clothing you can remove if you start getting too warm. In hot weather, protect yourself against the sun and heat.

- Warm up by walking more slowly for the first few minutes. Cool down by slowing your pace.

Dancing

Dancing can be a lot of fun while it tones your muscles, strengthens your heart and lungs, and boosts your mood. You can dance at a health club, dance studio, or even at home. Just turn on some lively music and start moving. You also can dance to a video on your TV or computer.

If you have trouble standing on your feet for a long time, try dancing while sitting down. Chair dancing lets you move your arms and legs to music while taking the weight off your feet.

Bicycling

Riding a bicycle spreads your weight among your arms, back, and hips. For outdoor biking, you may want to try a mountain bike. Mountain bikes have wider tires and are sturdier than bikes with thinner tires. You can buy a larger seat to make biking more comfortable.

For indoor biking, you may want to try a recumbent bike. On this type of bike, you sit lower to the ground with your legs reaching forward to the pedals. Your body is in more of a reclining position, which may feel better than sitting straight up. The seat on a recumbent bike is also wider than the seat on a regular bike. If you decide to buy a bike, check how much weight it can support to make sure it is safe for you.

Workout Clothing Tips

- Clothes made of fabrics that absorb sweat are best for working out.
- Comfortable, lightweight clothes allow you to move more easily.
- Tights or spandex shorts are the best bottoms to wear to prevent inner-thigh chafing.
- Women should wear a bra that provides extra support during physical activity.

Water Workouts

Swimming and water workouts put less stress on your joints than walking, dancing, or biking. If your feet, back, or joints hurt when you stand, water activities may be best for you. If you feel self-conscious about wearing a bathing suit, you can wear shorts and a T-shirt while you swim.

Exercising in water:

- Lets you be more flexible. You can move your body in water in ways you may not be able to on land.

- Reduces your risk of hurting yourself. Water provides a natural cushion, which keeps you from pounding or jarring your joints.

- Helps prevent sore muscles.

- Keeps you cool, even when you are working hard.

You don't need to know how to swim to work out in water. You can do shallow- or deep-water exercises at either end of the pool without swimming. For instance, you can do laps while holding onto a kickboard and kicking your feet. You also can walk or jog across the width of the pool while moving your arms.

For shallow-water workouts, the water level should be between your waist and chest. During deep-water workouts, most of your body is underwater. For safety and comfort, wear a foam belt or life jacket.

Tips For protecting Your Hair

If you're worried that pool water will damage or mess up your hair, try these tips:

- Use a swim cap to help protect your hair from pool chemicals and getting wet.
- Wear a natural hairstyle, short braids, locs, or twists, which may be easier to style after a water workout.
- Buy a shampoo to remove chlorine buildup, available at most drug stores, if your hair feels dry or damaged after a pool workout.

Strength Training

Strength training involves using free weights, weightlifting machines, resistance bands, or your own body weight to make your muscles stronger. Lower-body strength training will improve your balance and prevent falls.

Strength training may help you:

- build and maintain strong muscles as you get older

- continue to perform activities of daily living, such as carrying groceries or moving furniture

- keep your bones strong, which may help prevent osteoporosis and fractures

If you are just starting out, using a weightlifting machine may be safer than dumbbells. As you get fit, you may want to add free-weight exercises with dumbbells.

You do not need a weight bench or large dumbbells to do strength training at home. You can use a pair of hand weights to do bicep curls. You can also use your own body weight: for example, get up and down from a chair.

Strength-Training Tips

- Aim for 2 to 3 days per week of strength-training activities.
- Try to perform each exercise 8 to 12 times. If that's too hard, the weight you are lifting is too heavy. If it's too easy, your weight is too light.
- Try to exercise all the major muscle groups. These groups include the muscles of the legs, hips, chest, back, abdomen, shoulders, and arms.
- Don't work the same muscles 2 days in a row. Your muscles need time to recover.

Proper form is very important when lifting weights. You may hurt yourself if you don't lift weights properly. You may want to schedule a session with a certified fitness professional to learn which exercises to do and how to do them safely. Check with your health insurer about whether your health plan covers these services.

If you decide to buy a home gym, check how much weight it can support to make sure it is safe for you.

Mind And Body Exercise

Your local hospital or fitness, recreation, or community center may offer classes such as yoga, tai chi, or pilates. You also may find some of these workouts online and can download them to a computer, smartphone, or other device. These types of activities may help you:

- become stronger and more flexible

- feel more relaxed

- improve balance and posture

These classes also can be a lot of fun and add variety to your workout routine. If some movements are hard to do or you have injuries you are concerned about, talk with the instructor about how to adapt the exercises and poses to meet your needs—or start with a beginner's class.

Daily Life Activities

Daily life activities, such as cleaning out the attic or washing the car, are great ways to get moving. Small changes can add more physical activity to your day and improve your health. Try these:

- Take 2- to 3-minute walking breaks at work several times a day, if possible.
- Stand, walk, or stretch in place during TV commercials.
- Take the stairs instead of the elevator or escalator whenever you can.
- Park farther from where you are going and walk the rest of the way.

Even a shopping trip can be exercise because it provides a chance to walk and carry your bags. Chores such as mowing the lawn, raking leaves, and gardening also count.

Where Can I Be Active?

You can find many fun places to be active. Having more than one place may keep you from getting bored. Here are some options:

- Join or take a class at a local fitness, recreation, or community center.

- Enjoy the outdoors by taking a hike or going for a walk in a safe local park, neighborhood, or mall.

- Work out in the comfort of your own home with a workout video or by finding a fitness channel on your TV, tablet, or other mobile device.

Tips For Choosing A Fitness Center

- Make sure the center has exercise equipment for people who weigh more and staff to show you how to use it.

- Ask if the center has any special classes for people just starting out, or people with mobility or health issues.

- See if you can try out the center or take a class before you join.

- Try to find a center close to work or home. The quicker and easier the center is to get to, the better your chances of using it often.

- Make sure you understand the rules for joining and ending your membership, what your membership fee covers, any related costs, and the days and hours of operation.

How Can I Get Past My Roadblocks?

You most likely will face roadblocks that keep you from meeting your physical activity goals. Think about what keeps you from being active, then try to come up with creative ways to address those roadblocks.

Table 51.1. Getting Over The Barrier

Barrier	Solution
I don't have enough time.	Instead of doing one long workout session, build in three 10-minute bursts of activity during your day, such as a brisk walk. Even standing up instead of sitting at your desk has benefits.
I just don't like exercise.	Good news! You don't have to run a marathon or go to the gym all the time to benefit from being active. To make physical activity more fun, try something you enjoy doing, such as dancing to the radio or taking a yoga class with friends. Many people find they start to like exercise better the more they do it.

Table 51.1. Continued

Barrier	Solution
I'm worried about my health or getting hurt.	If you have a hard time being active because of your health, talk with a healthcare professional first. A certified fitness professional can also guide you on how to be active safely.
I feel self-conscious working out in front of others.	Start being active at home until you feel more confident. Be active with friends who will support and encourage you.

Chapter 52

Sports Injuries

What Are Sports Injuries?[1]

"Sports injuries" are injuries that happen when playing sports or exercising. Some are from accidents. Others can result from poor training practices or improper gear. Some people get injured when they are not in proper condition. Not warming up or stretching enough before you play or exercise can also lead to injuries. The most common sports injuries are:

- Sprains and strains

- Knee injuries

- Swollen muscles

- Achilles tendon injuries

- Pain along the shin bone

- Fractures

- Dislocations

Childhood Sports Injuries: A Common And Serious Problem[2]

Although sports participation provides numerous physical and social benefits, it also has a downside: the risk of sports-related injuries. According to the Centers for Disease Control

About This Chapter: This chapter includes text excerpted from documents published by two public domain sources. Text under headings marked 1 are excerpted from "Sports Injuries—Fast Facts About Sports Injuries," National Institute of Arthritis and Musculoskeletal and Skin Diseases (NIAMS), November 2014. Reviewed September 2017; Text under the headings marked 2 are excerpted from "Sports Injuries—Childhood Sports Injuries And Their Prevention: A Guide For Parents With Ideas For Kids," National Institute of Arthritis and Musculoskeletal and Skin Diseases (NIAMS), September 2016.

and Prevention (CDC), more than 2.6 million children 0 to 19 years old are treated in the emergency department each year for sports and recreation-related injuries.

These injuries are by far the most common cause of musculoskeletal injuries in children treated in emergency departments. They are also the single most common cause of injury-related primary care office visits.

The Most Common Musculoskeletal Sports-Related Injuries In Kids[1]

Although sports injuries can range from scrapes and bruises to serious brain and spinal cord injuries, most fall somewhere between the two extremes. Here are some of the more common types of injuries.

Sprains And Strains

A sprain is an injury to a ligament, one of the bands of tough, fibrous tissue that connects two or more bones at a joint and prevents excessive movement of the joint. An ankle sprain is the most common athletic injury.

A strain is an injury to either a muscle or a tendon. A muscle is a tissue composed of bundles of specialized cells that, when stimulated by nerve messages, contract and produce movement. A tendon is a tough, fibrous cord of tissue that connects muscle to bone. Muscles in any part of the body can be injured.

Growth Plate Injuries

In some sports accidents and injuries, the growth plate may be injured. The growth plate is the area of developing tissues at the end of the long bones in growing children and adolescents. When growth is complete, sometime during adolescence, the growth plate is replaced by solid bone. The long bones in the body include:

- the long bones of the hand and fingers (metacarpals and phalanges)
- both bones of the forearm (radius and ulna)
- the bone of the upper leg (femur)
- the lower leg bones (tibia and fibula)
- the foot bones (metatarsals and phalanges).

If any of these areas becomes injured, it's important to seek professional help from an orthopaedic surgeon, a doctor who specializes in bone injuries.

Repetitive Motion Injuries

Painful injuries such as stress fractures (a hairline fracture of the bone that has been subjected to repeated stress) and tendinitis (inflammation of a tendon) can occur from overuse of muscles and tendons. Some of these injuries don't always show up on X-rays, but they do cause pain and discomfort. The injured area usually responds to rest, ice, compression, and elevation (RICE). Other treatments can include crutches, cast immobilization, and physical therapy.

Preventing And Treating Musculoskeletal Injuries[2]

Injuries can happen to any child who plays sports, but there are some things that can help prevent and treat injuries.

Prevention

- Enroll your child in organized sports through schools, community clubs, and recreation areas that are properly maintained. Any organized team activity should demonstrate a commitment to injury prevention. Coaches should be trained in first aid and cardio-pulmonary resuscitation (CPR), and should have a plan for responding to emergencies. Coaches should be well versed in the proper use of equipment, and should enforce rules on equipment use.

- Organized sports programs may have people on staff who are certified athletic trainers. These individuals are trained to prevent, recognize, and provide immediate care for athletic injuries.

- Make sure your child has—and consistently uses—proper gear for a particular sport. This may reduce the chances of being injured.

- Make warm-ups and cool-downs part of your child's routine before and after sports participation. Warm-up exercises make the body's tissues warmer and more flexible. Cool-down exercises loosen muscles that have tightened during exercise.

- Make sure your child has access to water or a sports drink while playing. Encourage him or her to drink frequently and stay properly hydrated. Remember to include sunscreen and a hat (when possible) to reduce the chance of sunburn, which is a type of injury to the skin. Sun protection may also decrease the chances of malignant melanoma—a potentially deadly skin cancer—or other skin cancers that can occur later in life.

- Learn and follow safety rules and suggestions for your child's particular sport. You'll find some more sport-specific safety suggestions below.

Treatment

Treatment for sports-related injuries will vary by injury. But if your child suffers a soft tissue injury (such as a sprain or strain) or a bone injury, the best immediate treatment is easy to remember: RICE (rest, ice, compression, elevation) the injury. Get professional treatment if any injury is severe. A severe injury means having an obvious fracture or dislocation of a joint, prolonged swelling, or prolonged or severe pain.

Keep Kids Exercising[2]

It's important that kids continue some type of regular exercise after the injury heals. Exercise may reduce their chances of obesity, which has become more common in children. It may also reduce the risk of diabetes, a disease that can be associated with a lack of exercise and poor eating habits. Exercise also helps build social skills and provides a general sense of well-being. Sports participation is an important part of learning how to build team skills.

As a parent, it is important for you to encourage your children to be physically active. It's also important to match your child to the sport, and not push him or her too hard into an activity that he or she may not like or be capable of doing. Teach your children to follow the rules and to play it safe when they get involved in sports, so they'll spend more time having fun in the game and be less likely to be sidelined with an injury. You should be mindful of the risks associated with different sports and take important measures to reduce the chance of injury. For sport-specific suggestions, see the following information below.

Sport-Specific Safety Information[2]

Here are some winning ways to help prevent an injury from occurring.

Basketball

- **Common injuries and locations:** Sprains, strains, bruises, fractures, scrapes, dislocations, cuts, injuries to teeth, ankles, and knees. (Injury rates are higher in girls, especially for the anterior cruciate ligament or ACL, the wide ligament that limits rotation and forward movement of the shin bone.)

- **Safest playing with:** Eye protection, elbow and knee pads, mouth guard, athletic supporters for males, proper shoes, water. If playing outdoors, wear sunscreen and, when possible, a hat.

- **Injury prevention:** Strength training (particularly knees and shoulders), aerobics (exercises that develop the strength and endurance of heart and lungs), warm-up exercises, proper coaching, use of safety equipment.

Track And Field

- **Common injuries:** Strains, sprains, scrapes from falls.

- **Safest playing with:** Proper shoes, athletic supporters for males, sunscreen, water.

- **Injury prevention:** Proper conditioning and coaching.

Football

- **Common injuries and locations:** Bruises, sprains, strains, pulled muscles, tears to soft tissues such as ligaments, broken bones, internal injuries (bruised or damaged organs), concussions, back injuries, sunburn. Knees and ankles are the most common injury sites.

- **Safest playing with:** Helmet, mouth guard, shoulder pads, athletic supporters for males, chest/rib pads, forearm, elbow, and thigh pads, shin guards, proper shoes, sunscreen, water.

- **Injury prevention:** Proper use of safety equipment, warm-up exercises, proper coaching techniques and conditioning.

Baseball And Softball

- **Common injuries:** Soft tissue strains, impact injuries that include fractures caused by sliding and being hit by a ball, sunburn.

- **Safest playing with:** Batting helmet; shin guards; elbow guards; athletic supporters for males; mouth guard; sunscreen; cleats; hat; detachable, "breakaway bases" rather than traditional, stationary ones.

- **Injury prevention:** Proper conditioning and warm-ups.

Soccer

- **Common injuries:** Bruises, cuts and scrapes, headaches, sunburn.

- **Safest playing with:** Shin guards, athletic supporters for males, cleats, sunscreen, water.

- **Injury prevention:** Aerobic conditioning and warm-ups, and—when age appropriate—proper training in "heading" (that is, using the head to strike or make a play with the ball).

Gymnastics

- **Common injuries:** Sprains and strains of soft tissues.

- **Safest playing with:** Athletic supporters for males, safety harness, joint supports (such as neoprene wraps), water.

- **Injury prevention:** Proper conditioning and warm-ups.

What Should I Do If I Get Injured?[1]

Never try to "work through" the pain of a sports injury. Stop playing or exercising when you feel pain. Playing or exercising more only causes more harm. Some injuries should be seen by a doctor right away. Others you can treat yourself.

Call a doctor when:

- The injury causes severe pain, swelling, or numbness

- You can't put any weight on the area

- An old injury hurts or aches

- An old injury swells

- The joint doesn't feel normal or feels unstable.

If you don't have any of these signs, it may be safe to treat the injury at home. If the pain or other symptoms get worse, you should call your doctor. Use the RICE (Rest, Ice, Compression, and Elevation) method to relieve pain, reduce swelling, and speed healing. Follow these four steps right after the injury occurs and do so for at least 48 hours:

- **Rest.** Reduce your regular activities. If you've injured your foot, ankle, or knee, take weight off of it. A crutch can help. If your right foot or ankle is injured, use the crutch on the left side. If your left foot or ankle is injured, use the crutch on the right side.

- **Ice.** Put an ice pack to the injured area for 20 minutes, four to eight times a day. You can use a cold pack or ice bag. You can also use a plastic bag filled with crushed ice and wrapped in a towel. Take the ice off after 20 minutes to avoid cold injury.

- **Compression.** Put even pressure (compression) on the injured area to help reduce swelling. You can use an elastic wrap, special boot, air cast, or splint. Ask your doctor which one is best for your injury.

- **Elevation.** Put the injured area on a pillow, at a level above your heart, to help reduce swelling.

How Are Sports Injuries Treated?[1]

Treatment often begins with the RICE method. Here are some other things your doctor may do to treat your sports injury.

Nonsteroidal Anti-Inflammatory Drugs (NSAIDs)

Your doctor may suggest that you take a nonsteroidal anti-inflammatory drug (NSAID) such as aspirin or ibuprofen. These drugs reduce swelling and pain. You can buy them at a drug store. Another common drug is acetaminophen. It may relieve pain, but it will not reduce swelling.

Immobilization

Immobilization is a common treatment for sports injuries. It keeps the injured area from moving and prevents more damage. Slings, splints, casts, and leg immobilizers are used to immobilize sports injuries.

Surgery

In some cases, surgery is needed to fix sports injuries. Surgery can fix torn tendons and ligaments or put broken bones back in place. Most sports injuries don't need surgery.

Rehabilitation (Exercise)

Rehabilitation is a key part of treatment. It involves exercises that step by step get the injured area back to normal. Moving the injured area helps it to heal. The sooner this is done, the better. Exercises start by gently moving the injured body part through a range of motions. The next step is to stretch. After a while, weights may be used to strengthen the injured area.

As injury heals, scar tissue forms. After a while, the scar tissue shrinks. This shrinking brings the injured tissues back together. When this happens, the injured area becomes tight or stiff. This is when you are at greatest risk of injuring the area again. You should stretch the muscles every day. You should always stretch as a warmup before you play or exercise.

Don't play your sport until you are sure you can stretch the injured area without pain, swelling, or stiffness. When you start playing again, start slowly. Build up step by step to full speed.

Rest

Although it is good to start moving the injured area as soon as possible, you must also take time to rest after an injury. All injuries need time to heal; proper rest helps the process. Your doctor can guide you on the proper balance between rest and rehabilitation.

Other Therapies

Other therapies include mild electrical currents (electrostimulation), cold packs (cryotherapy), heat packs (thermotherapy), sound waves (ultrasound), and massage.

Chapter 53

Exercise Suggestions For People With Asthma

Who Has Asthma?

Asthma—which makes it hard to breathe, and causes coughing and wheezing—affects about five million American kids and teens?

That's almost 1 in 10!

Famous people like rapper Coolio have asthma, although he's better known for his hit songs like "Gangsta's Paradise" than for his fight against the illness.

Physical Activity And Asthma

Things like cold or dry air, dust, pollen, pollution, cigarette smoke, or stress can "trigger" asthma. This can make your body pump out chemicals that close off your airways, making it hard for air to get into to your lungs, and causing an asthma attack.

Physical activity can trigger asthma attacks too. Experts don't know for sure why physical activity sometimes brings one on, but they suspect that fast breathing through the mouth (like what happens when you get winded) can irritate the airways. In addition, when air pollution levels are high, physical activity in the afternoon is harder on the lungs than morning activity—pollution levels rise later in the day.

About This Chapter: This chapter includes text excerpted from "BAM! Body And Mind—Meeting The Challenge," Centers for Disease Control and Prevention (CDC), May 9, 2015.

Get Fit

So, should you get a doctor's note and skip gym class? Sorry, no. Doctors want their asthma patients to get active, especially in asthma-friendly activities like these: Swimming, bicycling, golf, inline skating, and weightlifting.

Why Are These Good Choices If You Want To Be Physically Active?

- They let you control how hard and fast you breathe

- They let you breathe through your nose at all times

- They don't dry out your airways

- They mix short, intense activities with long endurance workouts

- You can do them in a controlled environment (for example, a gym with air that's not too cold or dry)

- Usually you do them with other people, who can help you if an attack comes on

Getting regular physical activity can improve your breathing, and lead to fewer asthma attacks. Just remember to follow these tips. (In fact, this is good advice for everyone, not just those with asthma.)

- **Ease into it.**

  Start your workout with a warm-up, and don't overdo it by running five miles on your first day if you get winded walking around the block! Finish up with a cool-down.

- **Take a buddy.**

  It's more fun and a friend can help if you get into trouble.

- **Respect your body.**

  Stay away from the things that trigger your asthma. Help out your airways by breathing through your nose instead of your mouth. Take it easy on days when your asthma symptoms are really bugging you. And stick to the medicine routine that your doctor has set up.

- **Take breaks.**

  Treat yourself to rest and drink plenty of water.

- **Mix it up.**

For example, try going inline skating one day and taking a long walk the next.

Feel Good

To feel your best, do the right stuff to control your asthma. And listen to your doctors—they're on your team!

Dr. Asthma says that people with asthma "should expect to live a life that really isn't affected by asthma, except for having to follow the directions." He also says to speak up if you are having symptoms, and remember to "keep a good attitude and keep working to control the disease."

So, get out there and get moving! With good habits and today's medicines, you can go for the gold—or just join your friends on the basketball court, in the pool, on the dance floor.

Chapter 54

Exercise Suggestions For People With Diabetes

How Can Physical Activity Help Me Take Care Of My Diabetes?

Physical activity and keeping a healthy weight can help you take care of your diabetes and prevent diabetes problems. Physical activity helps your blood glucose, also called blood sugar, stay in your target range.

Physical activity also helps the hormone insulin absorb glucose into all your body's cells, including your muscles, for energy. Muscles use glucose better than fat does. Building and using muscle through physical activity can help prevent high blood glucose. If your body doesn't make enough insulin, or if the insulin doesn't work the way it should, the body's cells don't use glucose. Your blood glucose levels then get too high, causing diabetes.

Starting a physical activity program can help you lose weight or keep a healthy weight and keep your blood glucose levels on target. Even without reaching a healthy weight, just a 10 or 15 pound weight loss makes a difference in reducing the risk of diabetes problems.

Among people of all ages, 2015 data indicated the following:

- An estimated 23.1 million people—or 7.2 percent of the U.S. population—had diagnosed diabetes. This total included:
  - 132,000 children and adolescents younger than age 18 years (0.18% of the total U.S. population younger than age 18 years).

About This Chapter: This chapter includes text excerpted from "Diabetes And Physical Activity," National Institute of Diabetes and Digestive and Kidney Diseases (NIDDK), August 2014. Reviewed September 2017.

- 193,000 children and adolescents younger than age 20 years (0.24% of the total U.S. population younger than age 20 years).
- About 5 percent of people with diabetes are estimated to have type 1 diabetes.

(Source: "National Diabetes Statistics Report, 2017," Centers for Disease Control and Prevention (CDC).)

What Should I Do Before I Start A Physical Activity Program?

Before you start a physical activity program, you should:

- talk with your healthcare team

- plan ahead

- find an exercise buddy

- decide how you'll track your physical activity

- decide how you'll reward yourself

Talk with your healthcare team. Your healthcare team may include a doctor, nurse, dietitian, diabetes educator, and others. Always talk with your healthcare team before you start a new physical activity program. Your healthcare team will tell you a target range for your blood glucose levels.

People with diabetes who take insulin or certain diabetes medicines are more likely to have low blood glucose, also called hypoglycemia. If your blood glucose levels drop too low, you could pass out, have a seizure, or go into a coma. Physical activity can make hypoglycemia more likely or worse in people who take insulin or certain diabetes medicines, so planning ahead is key. It's important to stay active. Ask your healthcare team how to stay active safely.

Physical activity works together with healthy eating and diabetes medicines to prevent diabetes problems. Studies show that people with type 2 diabetes who lose weight with physical activity and make healthy changes to their eating plan are less likely to need diabetes and heart medicines. Ask your healthcare team about your healthy eating plan and all your medicines. Ask if you need to change the amount of medicine you take or the food you eat before any physical activity.

Plan ahead. Decide in advance what type of physical activity you'll do. Before you start, also choose:

- the days and times you'll be physically active

- the length of each physical activity session

- your plan for warming up, stretching, and cooling down for each physical activity session

- a backup plan, such as where you'll walk if the weather is bad

- how you will measure your progress

To make sure you stay active, find activities you like to do. If you keep finding excuses not to be physically active, think about why:

- Are your goals realistic?

- Do you need a change in activity?

- Would another time be more convenient?

Find an exercise buddy. Many people find they are more likely to be physically active if someone joins them. Ask a friend or family member to be your exercise buddy. When you do physical activities with a buddy you may find that you:

- enjoy the company

- stick to the physical activity plan

- are more eager to do physical activities

Being active with your family may help everyone stay at a healthy weight. Keeping a healthy weight may prevent them from developing diabetes or prediabetes. Prediabetes is when the amount of glucose in your blood is above normal yet not high enough to be called diabetes.

Decide how you'll track your physical activity. Write down your blood glucose levels and when and how long you are physically active in a record book. You'll be able to track your progress and see how physical activity affects your blood glucose. You can find tools to help track your daily activities at www.ndep.nih.gov.

Decide how you'll reward yourself. Reward yourself with a nonfood item or activity when you reach your goals. For example, treat yourself to a movie or buy a new plant for the garden.

How Do I Check My Blood Sugar?

You use a blood glucose meter to check your blood sugar. This device uses a small drop of blood from your finger to measure your blood sugar level. You can get the meter and supplies in a drug store or by mail.

Read the directions that come with your meter to learn how to check your blood sugar. Your healthcare team also can show you how to use your meter. Write the date, time, and result of the test in your blood sugar record. Take your blood sugar record and meter to each visit and talk about your results with your healthcare team.

People with diabetes have blood sugar targets that they try to reach at different times of the day. These targets are:

- Right before your meal: 80 to 130

- Two hours after the start of the meal: Below 180

(Source: "Know Your Blood Sugar Numbers: Use Them To Manage Your Diabetes," National Institute of Diabetes and Digestive and Kidney Diseases (NIDDK).)

What Kinds Of Physical Activity Can Help Me?

Many kinds of physical activity can help you take care of your diabetes. Even small amounts of physical activity can help. You can measure your physical activity level by how much effort you use.

Doctors suggest that you aim for 30 to 60 minutes of moderate to vigorous physical activity most days of the week. Children and adolescents with type 2 diabetes who are 10 to 17 years old should aim for 60 minutes of moderate to vigorous activity every day.

Your healthcare team can tell you more about what kind of physical activity is best for you. They can also tell you when and how much you can increase your physical activity level.

Light physical activity. Light activity is easy. Your physical activity level is light if you:

- are breathing normally

- are not sweating

- can talk normally or even sing

Moderate physical activity. Moderate activity feels somewhat hard. Your physical activity level is moderate if you:

- are breathing quickly, yet you're not out of breath

- are lightly sweating after about 10 minutes of activity

- can talk normally, yet you can't sing

Vigorous physical activity. Vigorous, or intense, activity feels hard. Your physical activity level is vigorous if you:

- are breathing deeply and quickly

- are sweating after a few minutes of activity

- can't talk normally without stopping for a breath

Not all physical activity has to take place at the same time. You might take a walk for 20 minutes, lift hand weights for 10 minutes, and walk up and down the stairs for 5 minutes.

Breaking the physical activity into different groups can help. You can:

Do Aerobic Exercise

Aerobic exercise is activity that uses large muscles, makes your heart beat faster, and makes you breathe harder. Doing moderate to vigorous aerobic exercise for 30 to 60 minutes a day most days of the week provides many benefits. You can even split up these minutes into several parts.

Talk with your healthcare team about how to warm-up and cool down before and after you exercise. Start slowly, with 5 to 10 minutes a day, and add a little more time each week. Try:

- walking briskly

- hiking

- climbing stairs

- swimming or taking a water-aerobics class

- dancing

- riding a bicycle outdoors or a stationary bicycle indoors

- taking an exercise class

- playing basketball, tennis, or other sports

- in-line skating, ice skating, or skateboarding

Do Strength Training To Build Muscle

Strength training is a light to moderate physical activity that builds muscle and keeps your bones healthy. When you have more muscle and less fat, you'll burn more calories because muscle burns more calories than fat, even between exercise sessions. Burning more calories can help you lose and keep off weight.

Whether you're a man or a woman, you can do strength training with hand weights, elastic bands, or weight machines two to three times a week. You can do strength training at home, at a fitness center, or in a class. Start with a light weight and slowly increase the size of your weights as your muscles become stronger.

Do Stretching Exercises

Stretching exercises are a light to moderate physical activity that both men and women can do. For example, yoga is a type of stretching that focuses on your breathing and helps you relax. Your healthcare team can suggest whether yoga is right for you.

Even if you have problems moving or balancing, certain types of yoga can help. For example, chair yoga has stretches you can do when sitting in a chair. When you stretch, you increase your flexibility, lower your stress, and help prevent sore muscles.

Add Extra Activity To Your Daily Routine

Increase daily activity by spending less time watching TV or at the computer. Try these simple ways to add light, moderate, or vigorous physical activities in your life every day:

- Walk around while you talk on the phone.

- If you have kids or grandkids, visit a zoo or a park with them.

- Take a walk through your neighborhood.

- When you watch TV, get up and walk around the room during commercials.

- Do chores, such as work in the garden or rake leaves, clean the house, or wash the car.

- Stretch out your chores. For example, make two trips to take the laundry downstairs instead of one.

- Park at the far end of the shopping center parking lot and walk to the store.

- Take the stairs instead of the elevator.

- Stretch or walk around instead of taking a coffee break and eating.

When Is The Best Time Of Day For Me To Do Physical Activity?

Your healthcare team can help you decide the best time of day for you to do physical activity based on your daily schedule, healthy eating plan, and diabetes medicines.

If you have type 1 diabetes, try not to do vigorous physical activity when you have ketones in your blood or urine. Ketones are chemicals your body might make when your blood glucose levels are too high and your insulin level is too low. If you are physically active when you have ketones in your blood or urine, your blood glucose levels may go even higher.

Light or moderate physical activity can help lower blood glucose if you have type 2 diabetes and you don't have ketones. Ketones are rare in people with type 2 diabetes. Ask your healthcare team whether you should be physically active when your blood glucose levels are high.

Points To Remember

- Starting a physical activity program can help you lose weight or keep a healthy weight and keep your blood glucose levels on target.

- Always talk with your healthcare team before you start a new physical activity program.

- Ask your healthcare team if you need to change the amount of medicine you take or the food you eat before any physical activity.

- Talk with your healthcare team about what types of physical activity are safe for you, such as walking, weight lifting, or housework.

- To make sure you stay active, find activities you like to do. Ask a friend or family member to be your exercise buddy.

- Write down your blood glucose levels and when and how long you are physically active in a record book.

- Doctors suggest that you aim for 30 to 60 minutes of moderate to vigorous physical activity most days of the week.

- Children and adolescents with type 2 diabetes who are 10 to 17 years old should aim for 60 minutes of moderate to vigorous activity every day.

- Not all physical activity has to take place at the same time. For example, you might take a walk for 20 minutes, lift hand weights for 10 minutes, and walk up and down the stairs for 5 minutes.

- Doing moderate to vigorous aerobic exercise for 30 to 60 minutes a day most days of the week provides many benefits. You can even split up these minutes into several parts.

- Start exercising slowly, with 5 to 10 minutes a day, and add a little more time each week. Try walking briskly, hiking, or climbing stairs.

- Whether you're a man or a woman, you can do strength training with hand weights, elastic bands, or weight machines two to three times a week.

- Stretching exercises are a light to moderate physical activity that both men and women can do. When you stretch, you increase your flexibility, lower your stress, and help prevent sore muscles.

- Increase daily activity by spending less time watching TV or at the computer.

- Try these simple ways to add light, moderate, or vigorous physical activities in your life every day:

  - Walk around while you talk on the phone.

  - Take a walk through your neighborhood.

  - Do chores, such as work in the garden or rake leaves, clean the house, or wash the car.

- If you have type 1 diabetes, try not to do vigorous physical activity when you have ketones in your blood or urine.

Chapter 55

Overtraining Syndrome And Compulsive Exercise

Overtraining Syndrome[1]

Are you the type of athlete that has a need to always practice, weight lift, or do some kind of cardiovascular workout? Does your mind tell you that training and training and more training will make you feel better? Do you also tell yourself that rest or sitting around is bad for you? If you answered yes, you might have what is known as overtraining syndrome, "staleness," or "burnout."

Maintaining Body Weight

Try to maintain your body weight by balancing what you eat with physical activity. If you are sedentary, try to become more active. If you are already very active, try to continue the same level of activity as you age. More physical activity is better than less, and any is better than none. If your weight is not in the healthy range, try to reduce health risks through better eating and exercise habits. Take steps to keep your weight within the healthy range (neither too high nor too low). Have children's heights and weights checked regularly by a health professional.

(Source: "Balance The Food You Eat With Physical Activity—Maintain Or Improve Your Weight," U.S. Department of Health and Human Services (HHS).)

About This Chapter: This chapter includes text excerpted from documents published by two public domain sources. Text under headings marked 1 are excerpted from "Feeling 'Stale' From Overtraining," National Aeronautics and Space Administration (NASA), n.d. Reviewed September 2017; Text under heading marked 2 is excerpted from "Exercise And Bone Health For Women: The Skeletal Risk Of Overtraining," National Institute of Arthritis and Musculoskeletal and Skin Diseases (NIAMS), May 2016; Text beginning with the heading "What Is Compulsive Exercise?" is © 2018 Omnigraphics. Reviewed September 2017.

Risk Factors[1]

Overtraining occurs when there is a continuous, excessive overload of exercise without proper rest and proper nutrition. Many people fail to adapt to the stress sustained during high intensity training because they don't give their bodies enough time to adapt and recuperate. A poorly designed program consisting of a rapid increase in volume and intensity, consistently high volume training, and insufficient time for rest and recovery can lead to the body shutting down. Other factors that will increase your chances for developing overtraining syndrome are frequent competition, preexisting medical conditions, poor diet, environmental stress, and psychosocial stress.

The Skeletal Risk Of Overtraining In Female Athletes[2]

Girls and women who engage in rigorous exercise regimens or who try to lose weight by restricting their eating are at risk for these health problems. They may include serious athletes, "gym rats" (who spend considerable time and energy working out), and girls and women who believe "you can never be too thin."

Some athletes see amenorrhea (the absence of menstrual periods) as a sign of successful training. Others see it as a great answer to a monthly inconvenience. And some young women accept it blindly, not stopping to think of the consequences. But missing your periods is often a sign of decreased estrogen levels. And lower estrogen levels can lead to osteoporosis, a disease in which your bones become brittle and more likely to break. Usually, bones don't become brittle and break until women are much older. But some young women, especially those who exercise so much that their periods stop, develop brittle bones, and may start to have fractures at a very early age. Some 20-year-old female athletes have been said to have the bones of an 80-year-old woman. Even if bones don't break when you're young, low estrogen levels during the peak years of bone-building, the preteen and teen years, can affect bone density for the rest of your life. And studies show that bone growth lost during these years may never be regained. Broken bones don't just hurt—they can cause lasting physical malformations. Have you noticed that some older women and men have stooped postures? This is not a normal sign of aging. Fractures from osteoporosis have left their spines permanently altered.

Signs Of Burnout[1]

With all these factors and living in a world filled with stress, how do you know if you have this syndrome? There are many signs and symptoms with overtraining, but the primary element is the unpredicted drop in performance. A person can train and compete at the same level as they are use to, but they will have greater difficulty in maintaining the performance. Other signs and symptoms include excessive muscle fatigue, increased resting heart rate, trouble sleeping, depression, anxiety, increased weight loss, frequent injuries, and illnesses.

Treatment[1]

Overtraining syndrome is not something that is hard to treat. First off, it is always wise to consult a physician if it is suspected. This can rule out any disease or illness that can be caused by overtraining. Recovery will take at least two weeks depending on how severe the case is. Your activities should be extremely limited, if not discontinued during this time frame, and proper rest and nutrition should be given. A diet of low fat and high carbohydrates is recommended because of the depleted glycogen level over the period of time.

Prevention[1]

Early recognition will prevent any damages that could affect the body. To prevent overtraining from occurring, have an alternative workout schedule with proper rest for the body in between. Training should alternate from a heavy workday to a light workday. Good nutrition complete with complex carbohydrates, fruits, vegetables, and protein should be part of the diet. Proper hydration is a must! A person exercising should take in at least 8 servings, 12 fluid ounce. each, of water per pound lost. Increases in training should be progressed slowly so the body has time to adapt. To increase in training, one should use the 10 percent rule. The 10 percent rule is an increase of 10 percent in either intensity, duration or volume in one workout session at a time. Intensity, duration, and volume should not be increased at the same time. Most importantly, educating yourself about proper exercise is a key. And listen to your body... It will tell you when it's had enough!

What Is Compulsive Exercise?

Compulsive exercise (also known as anorexia athletica) is a type of addiction in which a person feels that they must work out frequently, often several times a day, and feels anxious and guilty if they don't work out enough. For those struggling with a compulsive exercise disorder, working out is not a choice. Exercise becomes an obligation, one that takes over the person's life to an extreme degree. Working out becomes the most important priority, often at the expense of other activities. A person with compulsive exercise disorder will strive to work out even with an injury or illness that would normally prevent physical exertion. For this reason, compulsive exercise often creates severe physical and psychological problems.

Over-Exercising

Too much of a good thing can be very bad for you. Just like eating disorders, societal pressures to be thin can also push women to exercise too much. Over-exercise is when someone engages in strenuous physical activity to the point that is unsafe and unhealthy. In fact, some studies indicate that young women who are compelled to exercise at excessive levels are at risk for developing eating disorders.

Eating disorders and over-exercising go hand-in-hand—they both can be a result of an unhealthy obsession with your body. The most dangerous aspect of over-exercising is the ease with which it can go unrecognized. The condition can be easily hidden by an emphasis on fitness or a desire to be healthy. Like bulimia and anorexia, in which persons deny themselves adequate nutrition by restrictive eating behaviors, over-exercising is a controlled behavior that denies the body the energy and nutrition needed to maintain a healthy weight.

(Source: "Body Image," Office on Women's Health (OWH), U.S. Department of Health and Human Services (HHS).)

Research has shown that the majority of people with compulsive exercise disorder are female. Many people exercise compulsively in order to feel more in control of their lives, and they define their self-worth through athletic achievements. Some use exercise as a way to try to handle difficult emotions or depression, believing that physical exhaustion will eliminate negative feelings. Others develop compulsive exercise disorder through participation in competitive sports. External and internal pressure to succeed or excel in sports can drive an athlete to push workouts too far, too frequently. In these cases, exercise compulsion is driven by the belief that additional workouts will provide the edge needed to win.

Health Effects

Compulsive exercise is dangerous and can result in serious physical and psychological harm. Stress fractures can develop in weight-bearing areas of the body (such as feet and lower legs) as a result of repetitive, high-impact, weight-bearing activities such as running or jumping.

Stress fractures produce pain during exercise and can develop into more serious bone breaks if not allowed to heal properly.

Consider This

People who exercise compulsively often believe they are improving their health, but the negative effects of too much exercise can result in serious complications.

Damage to muscle and connective tissue is one common side effect of compulsive exercise. Fitness experts advocate for periods of rest between workouts to allow the body to heal from minor injuries and muscle strains. Long-term damage can result from insufficient rest time, including loss of muscle mass, particularly for those who also struggle with eating disorders. A malnourished body begins to break down muscle tissue for fuel when calories are not available to burn.

Low heart rate (bradycardia) is a condition that develops from metabolic disruptions due to over-exercising. The body's normal response to rapid weight loss is to slow the metabolism in an effort to burn as few calories as possible. Low heart rate typically results in low body temperature and decreased resting heart rate. Low heart rate can easily be mistaken as a positive result of exercise, but in cases of exercise compulsion, low heart rate can produce serious arrhythmias (irregular heart function) and even sudden death.

Osteoporosis results in bone loss which increases the risk of stress fractures. This is a particularly dangerous risk for those suffering from both compulsive exercise and eating disorders, due to malnutrition from a poor diet.

Amenorrhea is the loss of normal menstruation that often develops during rapid and severe weight loss. Amenorrhea can result in loss of bone density and other serious problems including reproductive issues.

Exercising to the point of exhaustion on a frequent basis overloads the body with adrenaline and cortisol hormones, which in turn compromise the body's natural immune system. This increases the likelihood of illness, fatigue, insomnia or other sleep-related problems, irritability, short attention span, and mood swings.

Did You Know?

Compulsive exercise can lead to other dangerous conditions such as bulimia, anorexia, obsessive-compulsive disorder, negative thinking, low self-esteem, and social isolation.

Signs And Symptoms Of Compulsive Exercise

Some of the warning signs of a compulsive exercise disorder include:

- Feeling guilty, anxious, or irritable about missing workouts

- Pushing yourself to exercise even when injured or ill

- Persistent exhaustion and fatigue

- Chronic insomnia or disrupted sleep

- Slower than normal heart rate

- Inability to rest or even to sit still

- Giving up social time with friends in order to work out

- Obsessive focus on the number of calories eaten and burned

- Constantly thinking about working out

- Working out even in bad weather

- Low body weight, being underweight for your height

- Feeling obligated to exercise

- Lack of enjoyment of physical activity

- Making up for eating by exercising more

- Lack of satisfaction from personal achievements, always feeling there is more to do

Treatment Of Compulsive Exercise

Treatment and recovery from compulsive exercise disorder can take months to years, depending on the individual person and situation. Some common treatment approaches include psychotherapy and medication to help manage compulsive disorders. Cognitive behavioral therapy can help to identify and correct negative thoughts and attitudes. Therapy can also help provide healthy strategies to address negative emotions, stress, low self-esteem and negative body image. Family therapy can be useful when external pressures to excel may have inadvertently caused a compulsive exercise disorder. Family members may not be aware of overly high expectations and the resulting stress that is placed on a young person. This can be particularly critical for athletes who participate in sports that emphasize being thin, such as ice skating, gymnastics, and dancing. Participating in these sports can create an unhealthy focus on body weight.

References

1. "Compulsive Exercise," The Nemours Foundation/KidsHealth®, October 2013.

2. "Compulsive Exercise: Are You Overdoing It?" WebMD, February 26, 2016.

3. "Exercise Compulsion and Its Dangers," Eating Disorder Hope, October 5, 2012.

Chapter 56

Female Athlete Triad: Three Symptoms That Mean Trouble

Being active is great. In fact, girls should be active at least an hour each day. Sometimes, though, a girl will be very active (such as running every day or playing a competitive sport), but not eat enough to fuel her activity. This can lead to health problems. What happens when girls don't eat enough to fuel their activity:

- A problem called "low energy availability"

- Period (menstrual) problems

- Bone problems

These three sometimes are called the female athlete triad. ("Triad" means a group of three.) They sometimes also are called Athletic Performance and Energy Deficit. (This means you have a "deficit," or lack, of the energy your body needs to stay healthy.)

A Problem Called "Low Energy Availability"

Your body needs healthy food to fuel the things it does, like fight infections, heal wounds, and grow. If you exercise, your body needs extra food for your workout. You can get learn how much food to eat based on your activity level using the SuperTracker tool (www.choosemy-plate.gov/MyPlate-Daily-Checklist).

"Energy availability" means the fuel from food that is not burned up by exercise and so is available for growing, healing, and more. If you exercise a lot and don't get enough nutrition,

About This Chapter: Text in this chapter begins with excerpts from "Do You Exercise A Lot?" girlshealth.gov, Office on Women's Health (OWH), March 27, 2015; Text under the heading "Amenorrheic Women And The Female Athlete Triad" is excerpted from "Calcium," Office of Dietary Supplements (ODS), National Institutes of Health (NIH), November 17, 2016.

you may have low energy availability. That means your body won't be as healthy and strong as it should be.

Some female athletes diet to lose weight. They may do this to qualify for their sport or because they think losing weight will help them perform better. But eating enough healthy food is key to having the strength you need to succeed. Also, your body needs good nutrition to make hormones that help with things like healthy periods and strong bones. Sometimes, girls may exercise too much and eat too little because they have an eating disorder. Eating disorders are serious and can even lead to death, but they are treatable.

Period (Menstrual) Problems

If you are very active, or if you just recently started getting your period (menstruating), you may skip a few periods. But if you work out really hard and do not eat enough, you may skip a lot of periods (or not get your period to begin with) because your body can't make enough of the hormone estrogen.

You may think you wouldn't mind missing your period, but not getting your period should be taken seriously. Not having your period can mean your body is not building enough bone, and the teenage years are the main time for building strong bones. If you have been getting your period regularly and then miss three periods in a row, see your doctor. Not having your period could be a sign of a serious health problem or of being pregnant. Also see your doctor if you are 15 years old and still have not gotten your period.

Bone Problems

Being physically active helps build strong bones. But you can hurt your bones if you don't eat enough healthy food to fuel all your activity. That's because your body won't be able to make the hormones needed to build strong bones.

One sign that your bones are weak is getting stress fractures, which are tiny cracks in bones. Some places you could get these cracks are your feet, legs, ribs, and spine.

Even if you don't have problems with your bones when you're young, not taking good care of them now can be a problem later in life. Your skeleton is almost completely formed by age 18, so it's important to build strong bones early in life. If you don't, then later on you could wind up with osteoporosis, which is a disease that makes it easier for bones to break.

Signs Of Not Eating Enough And Eating Disorders

Sometimes, girls exercise a lot and do not eat enough because they want to lose weight. Sometimes, exercising just lowers a person's appetite. And sometimes limiting food can be a sign that a girl may be developing an eating disorder. Here are some signs that you or a friend may have a problem:

- Worrying about gaining weight if you don't exercise enough

- Trying harder to find time to exercise than to eat

- Chewing gum or drinking water to cope with hunger

- Often wanting to exercise rather than be with friends

- Exercising instead of doing homework or other responsibilities

- Getting very upset if you miss a workout, but not if you miss a meal

- Having people tell you they are worried you are losing too much weight

If you think you or a friend has a problem, talk to a parent, guardian, or trusted adult.

Sometimes girls exercise a lot because they feel pressure to look a certain way. Soccer star Brandi Chastain knows how bad that can feel. It took a while, she says, for her to realize that only she was in charge of how she felt about her body. "Body image is tough, but it is something we have to take charge of," Brandi says. "Because inside, only we know who we are."

Amenorrheic Women And The Female Athlete Triad

Amenorrhea, the condition in which menstrual periods stop or fail to initiate in women of childbearing age, results from reduced circulating estrogen levels that, in turn, have a negative effect on calcium balance. Amenorrheic women with anorexia nervosa have decreased calcium absorption and higher urinary calcium excretion rates, as well as a lower rate of bone formation than healthy women. The "female athlete triad" refers to the combination of disordered eating, amenorrhea, and osteoporosis. Exercise-induced amenorrhea generally results in decreased bone mass. In female athletes and active women in the military, low bone-mineral density, menstrual irregularities, certain dietary patterns, and a history of prior stress fractures are associated with an increased risk of future stress fractures. Such women should be advised to consume adequate amounts of calcium and vitamin D. Supplements of these nutrients have been shown to reduce the risk of stress fractures in female Navy recruits during basic training.

Chapter 57

Steroids And Other Performance Enhancers Are Risky

Athletes want to win—sometimes taking extreme measures to push through the pain and perform at their best. But when has an athlete gone too far? When it gives the athlete an unfair advantage—and threatens his or her health.

Painless Play

Abusing drugs to overcome pain or inflate athletic abilities is definitely an unfair advantage. This doesn't include the appropriate use of doctor-prescribed treatments, such as cortisone injections or prescription opioid pain medications. However, using prescription pain medication in a way other than prescribed is not only unfair, it's dangerous. Besides causing confusion, nausea, and breathing problems, abuse of opioids can lead to addiction and overdose. Even abusing cortisone—which doesn't have the same medical risks as abusing opioids—can damage your joints.

Endless Endurance

Endurance is the ability to play or compete for a long time without needing a break. Athletes most often increase their endurance by exercising and training. However, some athletes turn to dishonest ways of increasing endurance such as blood doping, which boosts the number of red blood cells in the bloodstream. Because red blood cells carry oxygen from the lungs

About This Chapter: Text in this chapter begins with excerpts from "Crossing The Line: Athletes Risk Their Health When Using Performance-Enhancing Drugs," National Institute on Drug Abuse (NIDA) for Teens, December 11, 2014. Reviewed September 2017; Text beginning with the heading "What Are Anabolic Steroids?" is excerpted from "Anabolic Steroids," National Institute on Drug Abuse (NIDA), March 2016.

to the muscles, a higher concentration in the blood can improve an athlete's endurance. Many methods of blood doping are illegal, particularly in professional sports.

Famous athletes like Lance Armstrong and Alex Rodriguez have been linked to erythropoietin (EPO)—one method for blood doping. EPO is among the top two PEDs abused by athletes (the first being human growth hormone), even though it increases the risk for several deadly diseases such as heart disease, stroke, and a blood clot in the brain or lungs. Although blood doping can be difficult to detect, scientists are working on better methods of detection.

Pumped-Up Performance

Some athletes abuse performance-enhancing drugs (PEDs)—like anabolic steroids and stimulants (including caffeine and ephedrine, and even methamphetamine)—to help them perform better. Steroids build muscles and improve athletic performance. Stimulants increase focus, endurance, and speed. Each comes with its own set of risks. But in general, these PEDs increase the risk for high blood pressure, an enlarged heart, irregular heart rate, heart attack, stroke, dangerously high body temperatures, and intense anger or paranoia. Far from a winning combination!

What Are Anabolic Steroids?

Anabolic steroids are synthetic variations of the male sex hormone testosterone. The proper term for these compounds is anabolic-androgenic steroids. "Anabolic" refers to muscle building, and "androgenic" refers to increased male sex characteristics. Some common names for anabolic steroids are Gear, Juice, Roids, and Stackers. Healthcare providers can prescribe steroids to treat hormonal issues, such as delayed puberty. Steroids can also treat diseases that cause muscle loss, such as cancer and acquired immunodeficiency syndrome (AIDS). But some athletes and bodybuilders abuse these drugs to boost performance or improve their physical appearance.

How Do People Abuse Anabolic Steroids?

People who abuse anabolic steroids usually take them orally or inject them into the muscles. These doses may be 10 to 100 times higher than doses prescribed to treat medical conditions. Steroids are also applied to the skin as a cream, gel, or patch.

Some athletes and others who abuse steroids believe that they can avoid unwanted side effects or maximize the drugs' effects by taking them in ways that include:

- cycling—taking doses for a period of time, stopping for a time, and then restarting

- stacking—combining two or more different types of steroids

- pyramiding—slowly increasing the dose or frequency of abuse, reaching a peak amount, and then gradually tapering off

There is no scientific evidence that any of these practices reduce the harmful medical consequences of these drugs.

How Do Anabolic Steroids Affect The Brain?

Anabolic steroids work differently from other drugs of abuse; they do not have the same short-term effects on the brain. The most important difference is that steroids do not trigger rapid increases in the brain chemical dopamine, which causes the "high" that drives people to abuse other substances. However, long-term steroid abuse can act on some of the same brain pathways and chemicals—including dopamine, serotonin, and opioid systems—that are affected by other drugs. This may result in a significant effect on mood and behavior.

Short-Term Effects

Abuse of anabolic steroids may lead to mental problems, such as:

- paranoid (extreme, unreasonable) jealousy

- extreme irritability

- delusions—false beliefs or ideas

- impaired judgment

Extreme mood swings can also occur, including "roid rage"—angry feelings and behavior that may lead to violence.

What Are The Other Health Effects Of Anabolic Steroids?

Aside from mental problems, steroid use commonly causes severe acne. It also causes the body to swell, especially in the hands and feet.

Long-Term Effects

Anabolic steroid abuse may lead to serious, even permanent, health problems such as:

- kidney problems or failure

- liver damage

- enlarged heart, high blood pressure, and changes in blood cholesterol, all of which increase the risk of stroke and heart attack, even in young people

Several other effects are gender- and age-specific:

- In men:

- shrinking testicles

- decreased sperm count

- baldness

- development of breasts

- increased risk for prostate cancer

- In women:

- growth of facial hair or excess body hair

- male-pattern baldness

- changes in or stop in the menstrual cycle

- enlarged clitoris

- deepened voice

- In teens:

- stunted growth (when high hormone levels from steroids signal to the body to stop bone growth too early)

- stunted height (if teens use steroids before their growth spurt)

Some of these physical changes, such as shrinking sex organs in men, can add to mental side effects such as mood disorders.

Are Anabolic Steroids Addictive?

Even though anabolic steroids do not cause the same high as other drugs, they can lead to addiction. Studies have shown that animals will self-administer steroids when they have the chance, just as they do with other addictive drugs. People may continue to abuse steroids despite physical problems, high costs to buy the drugs, and negative effects on their relationships. These behaviors reflect steroids' addictive potential. Research has further found that some steroid users turn to other drugs, such as opioids, to reduce sleep problems and irritability caused by steroids.

People who abuse steroids may experience withdrawal symptoms when they don't use, including:

- mood swings

- fatigue

- restlessness

- loss of appetite

- sleep problems

- decreased sex drive

- steroid cravings

- One of the more serious withdrawal symptoms is depression, which can sometimes lead to suicide attempts.

How Can People Get Treatment For Anabolic Steroid Addiction?

Some people seeking treatment for anabolic steroid addiction have found behavioral therapy to be helpful. More research is needed to identify the most effective treatment options. In certain cases of severe addiction, patients have taken medicines to help treat symptoms of withdrawal. For example, healthcare providers have prescribed antidepressants to treat depression and pain medicines for headaches and muscle and joint pain. Other medicines have been used to help restore the patient's hormonal system.

Part Seven
Health And Wellness Trends

Chapter 58

Fitness And Exercise Trends

Physical fitness and exercise are two areas of modern life that are particularly subject to fluctuations in consumer interest. New fitness equipment and exercise programs catch the attention of those looking for the greatest results, replacing older approaches that have fallen out of favor. Some popular exercise programs quickly become fads, fading away after a brief period of widespread success in the fitness industry. Other fitness practices develop into trends, resulting in a more lasting change in the way people approach physical fitness. Some of the more popular current trends in fitness and exercise are described below.

Newer Trends

Wearable fitness trackers have become extremely popular among those with an interest in overall health and well-being. These portable devices use sensors and other technology to records various biometric data such as heart rate, and physical activities such as walking, running, stair climbing, and so on. Wearable fitness trackers often work in conjunction with smart phone apps or other web-enabled technology.

Functional fitness is a relatively new trend among fitness enthusiasts. Functional fitness refers to exercise that is performed to enhance one's ability to carry out tasks of daily living. Those who practice functional fitness generally seek to increase their strength, balance, coordination, and endurance in order to increase overall quality of life.

As the population of the U.S. ages, the popularity of fitness programs tailored specifically for older adults continues to grow. With the increase among senior citizens and retirees who are interested in continuing an active lifestyle, demand is increasing for fitness programs to serve this demographic.

High-intensity interval training (HIIT) is another popular fitness trend. This style of workout involves short periods of intense activity followed by short periods of rest. A high-intensity interval workout generally lasts about 30 minutes, although some sessions can run longer.

The use of special flexibility/mobility roller equipment is rising, particularly among those who experience issues with full range of motion. These rollers can be used during warm-up or cool-down periods, to work on areas of the body that are trigger points, or muscles that need focused attention or deep tissue work.

Weight Training

Strength training, also known as weightlifting or bodybuilding, is another somewhat timeless fitness trend that has never fallen out of favor. Strength training involves lifting weights, either free weights or through the use of weight-lifting machines, in a manner that targets specific muscles or groups of muscles. In strength training, various weights are lifted in repetitions known as sets, with periods of rest between sets. Strength training can be performed at a gym or at home, using traditional weights and/or weightlifting machines.

Bodyweight training, also known as calisthenics, is a minimalist form of exercise that requires no special equipment. Bodyweight training uses a person's own body mass as resistance, for example, exercises such as push-ups, sit-ups, and jumping jacks. This type of exercise was once the most popular form of physical training in the United States. Although it never completely fell out of favor, bodyweight training has at various times been eclipsed by newer activities and workouts based around gym equipment. Bodyweight training is experiencing a resurgence in popularity among those looking for a "back to basics" approach to fitness.

Personal Trainers, Fitness Coaches, And Wellness

Personal training continues to be a popular trend in fitness. Modern fitness enthusiasts are demanding fitness training services provided by educated, certified, experienced fitness professionals. Consumers of personal training services have become more aware of the benefits of working with a certified trainer, and many consumers look for trainers that have certain credentials or qualifications. Group personal training has gained popularity among those looking for a more cost-effective way to access the services of a personal trainer. In group personal training, a small group of people share the cost of personal training sessions. Under this arrangement, the personal trainer divides his or her time in the training session among all the group members. Online fitness training is another option that is growing in popularity among those who wish to access the services of a personal trainer at a time or place that is most convenient for them.

Wellness coaching is a form of personal fitness training that uses a more integrative approach to behavior modification. Wellness coaching often focuses on disease prevention, rehabilitation, and health maintenance. Sessions can occur in person, by phone or video, or other format, including individual one-on-one sessions or group meetings.

Wellness tourism is a relatively new trend among fitness enthusiasts. The term "wellness" encompasses the total state of a person's health, including physical, mental, and social aspects, with particular focus on proactive measures that promote, maintain, and improve one's overall healthiness. Wellness tourism, also known as fitness tourism, is any form of recreational travel that supports the goals of total personal wellness. Wellness tourism focuses on disease prevention and enhancement of healthy lifestyles through visits to spas, hot springs, and other therapeutic retreat centers.

Continuing Trends

Programs that combine exercise and weight loss continue to be popular choices for many fitness enthusiasts. These programs combine physical fitness coaching with nutrition and dietary instruction to promote a more rounded approach to health and well-being. Circuit training is another form of workout that has remained popular among fitness enthusiasts. Circuit training involves a selection of exercises that are done in sequence, normally to promote strength and endurance. One circuit is the completion of all the exercises in the program. Circuit training can include virtually any form of exercise, such as weightlifting, aerobics, and so on. Yoga remains one of the most popular and enduring fitness trends in recent years. Sometimes practiced for stress reduction and relaxation, yoga can also be a form of exercise centered on stretching the body and assuming specific poses for specific amounts of time.

References

1. Brown, Jill S. "Top Fitness Trends For 2016: Does Your Favorite Make The List?" Huffington Post, November 23, 2015.

2. Roberts. Amy. "Forecast: The Top 10 Fitness Trends In 2016," Men's Fitness, 2016.

3. Thompson, Walter R. "Worldwide Survey Of Fitness Trends For 2016: 10th Anniversary Edition," ACSM's Health and Fitness Journal, December 2015.

Chapter 59

Wellness Or Fitness Tourism

What Is Wellness Tourism?

The term "wellness" encompasses the total state of a person's health, including physical, mental, and social aspects, with particular focus on proactive measures that promote, maintain, and improve one's overall healthiness. Wellness tourism, also known as fitness tourism, is any form of recreational travel that supports the goals of total personal wellness. Wellness tourism focuses on disease prevention and enhancement of healthy lifestyles through visits to spas, hot springs, and other therapeutic retreat centers. In contrast, medical tourism addresses existing health problems through treatment at hospitals or other medical centers.

Types Of Wellness Tourism

There are many different types of wellness tourism opportunities that offer experiences and services addressing a broad spectrum of healthy living. Some wellness tourism destinations combine more than one area of focus, while others concentrate on a single aspect of overall health.

- **Eco Adventure:** Experiential destinations that typically emphasize time spent in nature, with activities such as hiking, biking, kayaking, paddle boarding, etc., and usually include guided tours. Some eco adventures include activities that are designed to be personally challenging, such as high ropes courses, extreme sports, or outdoor survival experiences.

- **Fitness:** Fitness retreats typically provide coaching and direction that emphasizes physical health, including gym workouts and other exercise programs such as pilates, stretching, cross-training, and so on. Some fitness retreats offer extreme sports activities or intensive boot-camp style physical programs.

- **Health:** These wellness tourism destinations typically focus on integrative health, often incorporating alternative medicine treatments, and therapies. Some health retreats focus on a specific issue such as stress management or relaxation techniques, while others promote overall health and well-being.

- **Healthy Eating:** Wellness centers that focus on healthy eating often provide instruction and guidance on nutrition, body cleansing and detoxification, organic eating, whole food diets, vegan or vegetarian living, weight management, and so on. Immersive weight-loss retreat centers typically combine nutrition and diet programs with fitness and exercise in a relaxed environment that fosters camaraderie among attendees.

- **Mind-Body:** These retreat centers often focus on wellness practices such as yoga, martial arts, meditation, tai chi, qigong, biofeedback, and so on.

- **Personal Growth and Development:** These lifestyle retreats often include activities intended to provide deep experiences of reflection and/or introspection through music, arts, writing, reading, life coaching, and so on.

- **Spa and Beauty:** Health resorts and specialty cruises provide a range of spa services including massage, therapeutic baths, hot springs, body treatments, facials, and other salon services.

- **Spiritual Connection:** Wellness centers that emphasize spiritual connection practices often include activities such as yoga, prayer, volunteering, time alone, time in silence, meditation, and so on.

Wellness Tourism Trends In The United States

Interest in wellness tourism is increasing in the United States, with billions of dollars being spent at these types of destinations each year. Wellness tourism is popular among people who strive for a healthy lifestyle and want to incorporate those habits and interests into their travel experiences. In general, wellness tourists seek out experiences and destinations that help them maintain healthy lifestyles, often through activities that promote rejuvenation and relaxation, meaning and connection to self or others, authentic experiences as opposed to traditional tourist activities, and opportunities to learn about disease prevention and maintenance of overall good health. Wellness tourists are generally categorized in two groups: primary purpose and secondary purpose.

Primary-purpose wellness tourists are those who travel to wellness tourism destinations such as those listed above. Primary-purpose wellness tourists choose a vacation destination specifically for the wellness programs, services, or experiences that are offered.

Secondary-purpose wellness tourists are those who partake of wellness-related activities as part of their travel, for example visiting a gym, spa, or wellness center while on vacation or a business trip. Secondary-purpose wellness tourists strive to maintain healthy lifestyles and general wellness while travelling for other purposes.

References

1. "The Global Wellness Tourism Economy Executive Summary," Global Wellness Institute, October 2013.

2. "Wellness Tourism, A US$500 Billion Travel Industry," The Yucatan Times, July 31, 2015.

3. "Wellness tourism: An Emerging Trend In Travel," Ontario Blue Cross, January 27, 2016.

Chapter 60

Online Fitness Training

What Is Online Fitness Training?

Online fitness training refers to the practice of working with a personal trainer or fitness coach via the Internet instead of in person. In most online fitness training programs, people subscribe to receive access to exercise programs and/or additional information and services from a personal trainer. Exercise programs are typically provided via video and are sometimes supplemented with written materials provided by e-mail, website, online chat, or other format.

General online fitness training usually consists of access to videos only. These videos contain recorded exercise routines to provide a virtual workout or exercise class experience, with no interaction between the instructor and the subscriber. Subscribers follow along with the video, performing the same moves shown on screen. In this format, the same videos are provided to all subscribers.

Personalized online fitness training often includes exercise programs and routines designed especially for the individual subscriber. This form of online fitness training generally includes some level of interactivity with the fitness trainer, which allows the consumer to ask questions and receive additional guidance.

Personalized online fitness training is sometimes offered in varying levels or packages. The most basic package might include a small monthly fee for access to online videos and website materials related to fitness, exercise, nutrition, or an online discussion area where subscribers share tips, personal experiences, and motivate each other. Another package might include more personalized information for a higher monthly fee. In this level, each subscriber typically has access to an individual trainer who provides exercise and nutrition plans and feedback tailored

"Online Fitness Training," © 2018 Omnigraphics. Reviewed September 2017.

to individual goals. Interaction between the trainer and the subscriber can be by phone, email, and/or webcam. At the highest service level, subscribers can often gain unlimited access to a personal trainer who works with them at every level, including assessment, goal setting, accountability, progression, and so on.

Are Online Training Programs Effective?

Online fitness training programs can be effective for subscribes who are self-motivated and able to commit to following a program on their own, without a trainer by their side during workouts. Advantages to online fitness training include:

- **Accessibility of personal trainers:** For those who travel often or live in an area without access to an experienced personal trainer.

- **Access to well-known trainers:** Online fitness training allows subscribers to benefit from working with a highly experienced trainer no matter where they are located.

- **Access to specialized trainers:** For those who want specialized training, online fitness training can be a way to work with established experts who are located in distant areas.

- **Reference checking:** Online fitness trainers often gain their reputation through client reviews, social media activity, and other online forums. Subscribers can thoroughly research an online trainer before engaging in a potentially costly relationship.

- **Lower cost of training:** An expert personal trainer has limited time to work with clients in person, and high demand can influence the cost of training sessions. In some cases, monthly subscription fees may be the same as a one-hour session of in-person training.

- **Flexibility:** Subscribers can access workouts at any convenient time and place.

- **Support:** Online trainers often provide more support options than in-person trainers through the use of email or other forms of communication.

Disadvantages Of Online Training Programs

There are also disadvantages to online fitness training programs. Some of these include:

- **Lack of personalization:** Some fitness programs are not personalized for an individual's goals, but intended to serve as many people as possible.

- **Lack of motivation:** Subscribers need to be able to motivate themselves without the trainer at their side during workouts.

- **Cost:** Even the lowest monthly fee can be a burden for some potential subscribers.

- **Lack of guidance on technique:** Without the trainer present during workouts, there is no immediate feedback or correction on exercise form, method, or performance.

- **Difficult to assess progress:** Online trainers sometimes have difficulty accurately measuring the progress of clients because the trainer is not present during workouts.

Is Online Training Right For You?

As with in-person fitness training, consumers should carefully evaluate the offerings, skills, and experience of any potential online fitness trainers. Some points to keep in mind include:

- Can an individual trainer help you meet your goals? Do their programs address your areas of concern? Look for a trainer who provides workouts that work for you.

- Is an individual trainer knowledgeable of current practices in health and fitness? What are their qualifications and experience?

- Can an individual trainer provide references from former or current clients? Can you verify that their programs produce results?

- Is an individual trainer reviewed or discussed online? Web searches can often provide insight on an individual trainer's reputation.

- Does an individual trainer offer something that you can't get on your own or through one or two sessions with an in-person trainer?

References

1. Laidler, Scott. "Does Online Personal Training Work?" The Telegraph, April 24, 2014.

2. "The Next Frontier Of Fitness: An Introduction To Online Personal Training," Bodybuilding.com, May 29, 2013.

3. Smith, Dave. "The 50 Best Free Workout Resources You Can Find Online," Huffington Post, June 7, 2016.

Chapter 61

Digital Health And Fitness Wearables

The broad scope of digital health includes categories such as mobile health (mHealth), health information technology (IT), wearable devices, telehealth and telemedicine, and personalized medicine.

Providers and other stakeholders are using digital health in their efforts to:

- Reduce inefficiencies
- Improve access
- Reduce costs
- Increase quality
- Make medicine more personalized for patients

Patients and consumers can use digital health to better manage and track their health and wellness related activities. The use of technologies such as smart phones, social networks and Internet applications is not only changing the way we communicate, but is also providing innovative ways for us to monitor our health and well-being and giving us greater access to

---

About This Chapter: Text in this chapter begins with excerpts from "Digital Health," U.S. Food and Drug Administration (FDA), September 6, 2017; Text beginning with the heading "Wearable Trackers" is excerpted from "A Comparison Of Wearable Fitness Devices," U.S. National Library of Medicine (NLM), National Institutes of Health (NIH), May 24, 2016; Text beginning with the heading "Ingestibles, Wearables And Embeddables" is excerpted from "Ingestibles, Wearables And Embeddables," Federal Communications Commission (FCC), January 30, 2015; Text beginning with the heading "Mobile Medical Apps" is excerpted from "Mobile Medical Applications," U.S. Food and Drug Administration (FDA), September 22, 2015.

information. Together these advancements are leading to a convergence of people, information, technology, and connectivity to improve healthcare and health outcomes.

Why Is The FDA Focusing On Digital Health?

Many medical devices now have the ability to connect to and communicate with other devices or systems. Devices that are already U.S. Food and Drug Administration (FDA) approved or cleared are being updated to add digital features. New types of devices that already have these capabilities are being explored.

Many stakeholders are involved in digital health activities, including patients, healthcare practitioners, researchers, traditional medical device industry firms, and firms new to FDA regulatory requirements, such as mobile application developers.

FDA's Center for Devices and Radiological Health (CDRH) is excited about these advances and the convergence of medical devices with connectivity and consumer technology.

The following are topics in the digital health field on which the FDA has been working to provide clarity using practical approaches that balance benefits and risks:

- Wireless Medical Devices
- Mobile medical apps
- Health IT
- Telemedicine
- Medical Device Data Systems
- Medical device Interoperability
- Software as a Medical Device (SaMD)
- General Wellness
- Cybersecurity

How Is The FDA Advancing Digital Health?

CDRH has established the Digital Health Program which seeks to better protect and promote public health and provide continued regulatory clarity by:

- Fostering collaborations and enhancing outreach to digital health customers
- Developing and implementing regulatory strategies and policies for digital health technologies

Wearable Trackers

Wearable trackers can help motivate you during workouts and provide information about your daily routine or fitness in combination with your smartphone without requiring potentially disruptive manual calculations or records. This paper summarizes and compares wearable fitness devices, also called "fitness trackers" or "activity trackers."

These devices are becoming increasingly popular in personal healthcare, motivating people to exercise more throughout the day without the need for lifestyle changes. The various choices in the market for wearable devices are also increasing, with customers searching for products that best suit their personal needs. Further, using a wearable device or fitness tracker can help people reach a fitness goal or finish line. Generally, companies display advertising for these kinds of products and depict them as beneficial, user friendly, and accurate. However, there are no objective research results to prove the veracity of their words. This research features subjective and objective experimental results, which reveal that some devices perform better than others.

Ingestibles, Wearables And Embeddables

Routine tests can be anything but. Appointment times are often inconvenient. You may be at the mercy of walk-in labs and testing facilities, where waiting could be uncertain and often longer than many people can accommodate. Personal health—which should be a top priority—can suffer when important diagnostic tests fall off our to-do lists.

Recent advances in broadband-enabled sensor technology offer the potential for the emergence of more convenient, ultimately less-costly—and less-invasive—solutions. For example, we may soon see wide-spread use of smart clothing (or smart "tattoo" applications) that use skin-based sensors to measure things like heart rate, respiration and blood pressure. These new types of technologies are generically called "ingestibles," "wearables" and "embeddables."

Ingestibles are broadband-enabled digital tools that we actually "eat." For example, there are "smart" pills that use wireless technology to help monitor internal reactions to medications. Or imagine a smart pill that tracks blood levels of medications in a patient's body throughout the day to help physicians find optimum dosage levels, avoid overmedicating, and truly individualize treatment. Also, miniature pill-shaped video cameras may one day soon replace colonoscopies or endoscopies. Patients would simply swallow a "pill," which would collect and transmit images as it makes its way through the digestive system.

Wearables are digital tools you can "wear," such as wristwatch-like devices that have sensors to monitor your heart rate and other vital signs. Beyond medical monitoring, such wearables may also help improve athletic performance, track fitness goals or help prevent dangerous falls in the elderly. In fact, designers are now able to put sensors in T-shirts and other clothing to monitor perspiration as a stress indicator. And, "tattoo-like" sensor that could be peeled off after use or that might be absorbed by the body are another similar advance. These sensors gather data through skin contact and transmit information wirelessly to smartphones and remote diagnostic facilities.

Embeddables are miniature devices that are actually inserted under the skin or deeper into the body. A heart pacemaker is one kind of embeddable device. In the future, embeddables may use nanotechnology and be so tiny that doctors would simply "inject" them into our bodies. Some promising applications in this area could help diabetes patients monitor their blood sugar levels reliably and automatically, without the need to prick their fingers or otherwise draw blood.

Part Eight
If You Need More Information

Chapter 62

The President's Challenge

The President's Challenge Physical Activity & Fitness Awards Program, a program of the President's Council on Fitness, Sports & Nutrition (PCFSN), recognized nearly 70 million Americans of all ages and ability levels for their physical activity and nutrition achievements since 1988. Through a variety of programs, including the longstanding and evolving youth fitness test, the President's Challenge provided tools and resources to motivate youth and adults to meet the *Physical Activity and Dietary Guidelines for Americans*.

On August 31, 2016, the programs that comprise the President's Challenge underwent an organizational transition to better serve the American public. New and existing partnerships are providing additional resources for these programs to improve their efficiency, accessibility, and physical activity and nutrition tracking options. As part of the transition, the President's Challenge office in Bloomington, Indiana, is closed.

Key Details On The Program Transitions

Presidential Youth Fitness Program (PYFP)

The Presidential Youth Fitness Program (PYFP) provides educators with the necessary tools and information to achieve excellence through quality fitness education and assessment practices. PYFP was launched in 2012 to phase out the Presidential Physical Fitness Test. This new program to assess student fitness levels now, provides additional tools and resources, to ensure students are fit for life. With an evolved approach, the fitness assessment has moved away from recognizing athletic fitness to providing a barometer on student's health.

About This Chapter: This chapter includes text excerpted from "Award Program Information," President's Council on Fitness, Sports & Nutrition (PCFSN), May 19, 2017.

PYFP operates through a public-private partnership between the PCFSN, the Centers for Disease Control and Prevention (CDC), the Cooper Institute, SHAPE America, and the National Fitness Foundation. All program resources and information about how to get involved can be found at pyfp.org.

PYFP Frequently Asked Questions

How Can I Order My Student Recognition Items For The Presidential Youth Fitness Program?

You can order your recognition items by visiting The Loyalist's award store www.theloyalist.com/pyfp or by calling 646-363-6896.

I Have A Question About My Order. Who Can I Contact?

The Loyalist is the award vendor for the Presidential Youth Fitness Program. Please contact The Loyalist directly at 646-363-6896 and/or pyfp@theloyalist.com.

I'm Still Using The Presidential, National, And Participant Awards From The Youth Fitness Test. How Does This Transition Affect Me?

These award items are no longer available. The Youth Fitness Test was sunset in 2013. All physical educators interested in assessing student fitness are encouraged to get started with the Presidential Youth Fitness Program (pyfp.org/how-it-works/get-started). New awards are available for PYFP.

Presidential Active Lifestyle Award (PALA+)

The PALA+ program is now part of the U.S. Department of Agriculture's (USDA) Super-Tracker—a free online tool for tracking daily food and physical activity. You can begin an eight-week PALA+ program at any time on SuperTracker or by using the PALA+ paper log.

Presidential Champions

The Presidential Champions program is now part of the USDA's SuperTracker—a free online tool for tracking daily food and physical activity. Individuals who participated in the program on the President's Challenge website before August 2016 can follow an easy two-step process to resume earning points towards awards, and the program is open to new sign-ups.

Chapter 63

Resources For More Information About Fitness

Government Agencies That Provide Information About Fitness And Exercise

Agency for Healthcare Research and Quality (AHRQ)

Office of Communications and Knowledge Transfer
5600 Fishers Ln.
Seventh Fl.
Rockville, MD 20857
Phone: 301-427-1364
Website: www.ahrq.gov

Americans with Disabilities Act (ADA)

U.S. Department of Justice (DOJ)
950 Pennsylvania Ave. N.W.
Washington, DC 20530
Toll-Free: 800-514-0301
Phone: 202-307-0663
Toll-Free TTY: 800-514-0383
Fax: 202-307-1197
Website: www.ada.gov/contact_drs.htm

About This Chapter: Resources in this chapter were compiled from several sources deemed reliable; all contact information was verified and updated in September 2017.

Centers for Disease Control and Prevention (CDC)
1600 Clifton Rd.
Atlanta, GA 30329-4027
Toll-Free: 800-CDC-INFO (800-232-4636)
Phone: 404-639-3311
Toll-Free TTY: 888-232-6348
Website: www.cdc.gov

Centers for Medicare and Medicaid Services (CMS)
7500 Security Blvd.
Baltimore, MD 21244
Toll-Free: 800-MEDICARE (800-633-4227)
Phone: 410-786-3000
Toll-Free TTY: 877-486-2048
Website: www.cms.gov

ChooseMyPlate.gov
USDA Center for Nutrition Policy and Promotion
3101 Park Center Dr.
Alexandria, VA 22302-1594
Website: www.choosemyplate.gov/contact

Food and Nutrition Information Center (FNIC)
USDA National Agricultural Library
10301 Baltimore Ave.
Beltsville, MD 20705
Phone: 301-504-5755
Fax: 301-504-7042
Website: www.nal.usda.gov/contact-us

Healthcare.gov
Website: www.healthcare.gov/contact-us

National Center for Complementary and Integrative Health (NCCIH)
9000 Rockville Pike
Bethesda, MD 20892
Toll-Free: 888-644-6226
TTY: 866-464-3615
Website: www.nccih.nih.gov/tools/contact.htm

National Eye Institute (NEI)

Information Office
31 Center Dr.
MSC 2510
Bethesda, MD 20892-2510
Phone: 301-496-5248
Website: www.nei.nih.gov
E-mail: 2020@nei.nih.gov

National Heart, Lung, and Blood Institute (NHLBI)

P.O. Box 30105
Bethesda, MD 20824-0105
Phone: 301-592-8573
Website: www.nhlbi.nih.gov
E-mail: nhlbiinfo@nhlbi.nih.gov

National Institute of Arthritis and Musculoskeletal and Skin Diseases (NIAMS)

1 AMS Cir.
Bethesda, MD 20892-3675
Toll-Free: 877-22-NIAMS (877-226-4267)
Phone: 301-495-4484
TTY: 301-565-2966
Fax: 301-718-6366
Website: www.niams.nih.gov
E-mail: NIAMSinfo@mail.nih.gov

National Institute of Dental and Craniofacial Research (NIDCR)

Bethesda, MD 20892-2190
Toll-Free: 866-232-4528
Phone: 301-496-4261
Website: www.nidcr.nih.gov
E-mail: nidcrinfo@mail.nih.gov

National Institute of Diabetes and Digestive and Kidney Diseases (NIDDK)

31 Center Dr. MSC 2560
Bldg. 31 Rm. 9A06
Bethesda, MD 20892-2560
Phone: 301-496-3583
Website: www.niddk.nih.gov

National Institute of Neurological Disorders and Stroke (NINDS)

P.O. Box 5801
Bethesda, MD 20824
Toll-Free: 800-352-9424
Phone: 301-496-5751
Website: www.ninds.nih.gov

National Institutes of Health (NIH)

9000 Rockville Pike
Bethesda, MD 20892
Phone: 301-496-4000
Website: www.nih.gov
E-mail: NIHinfo@od.nih.gov

Office of Dietary Supplements (ODS)

National Institutes of Health (NIH)
6100 Executive Blvd.
Rm. 3B01 MSC 7517
Bethesda, MD 20892-7517
Toll-Free: 888-723-3366
Phone: 301-435-2920
Fax: 301-480-1845
Website: www.ods.od.nih.gov
E-mail: ods@nih.gov

Office on Women's Health (OWH)

200 Independence Ave. S.W.
Rm. 712E
Washington, DC 20201
Toll-Free: 800-994-9662
Phone: 202-690-7650
Toll-Free TDD: 888-220-5446
Fax: 202-205-2631
Website: www.womenshealth.gov

President's Council on Fitness, Sports & Nutrition (PCFSN)

1101 Wootton Pkwy
Ste. 560
Rockville, MD 20852
Phone: 240-276-9567
Fax: 240-276-9860
Website: www.hhs.gov/fitness/about-pcfsn/contact-us/index.html
E-mail: fitness@hhs.gov

U.S. Consumer Product Safety Commission (CPSC)

4330 E.W. Hwy
Bethesda, MD 20814
Toll-Free: 800-638-2772
Phone: 301-504-7923
TTY: 301-595-7054
Fax: 301-504-0124; 301-504-0025
Website: www.cpsc.gov/About-CPSC/Contact-Information/

U.S. Department of Health and Human Services (HHS)

200 Independence Ave. S.W.
Washington, DC 20201
Toll-Free: 877-696-6775
Website: www.hhs.gov

U.S. Food and Drug Administration (FDA)

10903 New Hampshire Ave.
Silver Spring, MD 20993
Toll-Free: 888-INFO-FDA (888-463-6332)
Website: www.fda.gov

U.S. National Library of Medicine (NLM)

Reference and Web Services
8600 Rockville Pike
Bethesda, MD 20894
Toll-Free: 888-FIND-NLM (888-346-3656)
Phone: 301-594-5983
Toll-Free TDD: 800-735-2258
Fax: 301-402-1384
Website: www.nlm.nih.gov
E-mail: custserv@nlm.nih.gov

U.S. Public Health Service Commissioned Corps (PHSCC)

Toll-Free: 800-279-1605
Website: www.dcp.psc.gov/ccmis/contact_usphs.aspx
E-mail: Corpsrecruitment@hhs.gov

Weight-Control Information Network (WIN)

31 Center Dr.
Rm. 9A06 MSC 2560
Bethesda, MD 20892-2560
Toll-Free: 800–860–8747
Phone: 301-496-3583
Website: www.niddk.nih.gov
E-mail: healthinfo@niddk.nih.gov

Private Organizations That Provide Information About Fitness And Exercise

Academy for Sports Dentistry

118 Faye St.
P.O. Box 364
Farmersville, IL 62533
Toll-Free: 800-273-1788
Phone: 217-241-6747
Fax: 217-529-9120
Website: www.asd.memberclicks.net/about-us
E-mail: sportsdentistry@consolidated.net

Academy of Nutrition and Dietetics

120 S. Riverside Plaza
Ste. 2190
Chicago, IL 60606-6995
Toll-Free: 800-877-1600
Phone: 312-899-0040
Website: www.eatrightpro.org/resource/about-us/academy-vision-and-mission/who-we-are/contact-us
E-mail: knowledge@eatright.org

Action for Healthy Kids
600 W. Van Buren St.
Ste. 720
Chicago, IL 60607
Toll-Free: 800-416-5136
Fax: 312-212-0098
Website: www.actionforhealthykids.org/contact-us

Aerobics and Fitness Association of America (AFAA)
1750 E. Northrop Blvd.
Ste. 200
Chandler, AZ 85286-1744
Toll-Free: 800-446-2322
Website: www.afaa.com/contact

American Academy of Orthopaedic Surgeons (AAOS)
9400 W. Higgins Rd.
Rosemont, IL 60018
Phone: 847-823-7186
Fax: 847-823-8125
Website: www.aaos.org
E-mail: custserv@aaos.org

American Academy of Pediatrics (AAP)
141 N.W. Pt. Blvd.
Elk Grove Village, IL 60007-1098
Toll-Free: 800-433-9016
Phone: 847-434-4000
Fax: 847-434-8000
Website: www.aap.org/en-us/Pages/Contact.aspx

American Academy of Physical Medicine and Rehabilitation (AAPM&R)
9700 W. Bryn Mawr Ave.
Ste. 200
Rosemont, IL 60018
Phone: 847-737-6000
Website: www.aapmr.org
E-mail: info@aapmr.org

American Academy of Podiatric Sports Medicine (AAPSM)
3121 N.E. 26th St.
Ocala, FL 34470
Phone: 352-620-8562
Website: www.aapsm.org/inquiry.php
E-mail: info@aapsm.org

American Academy of Otolaryngology—Head and Neck Surgery (AAO-HNS)
1650 Diagonal Rd.
Alexandria, VA 22314-2857
Phone: 703-836-4444
Website: www.entnet.org/contact_us

American Association of Cardiovascular and Pulmonary Rehabilitation (AACVPR)
330 N. Wabash Ave.
Ste. 2000
Chicago, IL 60611
Phone: 312-321-5146
Fax: 312-673-6924
Website: www.aacvpr.org
E-mail: aacvpr@aacvpr.org

American Chiropractic Association (ACA)
1701 Clarendon Blvd., Ste. 200
Arlington, VA 22209
Phone: 703-276-8800
Fax: 703-243-2593
Website: www.acatoday.org/Contact-Us
E-mail: memberinfo@acatoday.org

American College of Cardiology (ACC)
Heart House
2400 N. St. N.W.
Washington, DC 20037
Toll-Free: 800-253-4636
Phone: 202-375-6000
Fax: 202-375-7000
Website: www.acc.org
E-mail: resource@aac.org

American College of Chest Physicians (ACCP)
3300 Dundee Rd.
Northbrook, IL 60062-2348
Toll-Free: 800-343-2227
Phone: 847-498-1400
Fax: 847-498-5460
Website: www.chestnet.org

American College of Rheumatology (ACR)
2200 Lake Blvd. N.E.
Atlanta, GA 30319
Phone: 404-633-3777
Fax: 404-633-1870
Website: www.rheumatology.org/Contact
E-mail: website@rheumatology.org

American College of Sports Medicine (ACSM)
401 W. Michigan St.
Indianapolis, IN 46202-3233
Phone: 317-637-9200
Fax: 317-634-7817
Website: www.acsm.org

American Council on Exercise (ACE)
4851 Paramount Dr.
San Diego, CA 92123
Toll-Free: 888-825-3636
Phone: 858-576-6500
Fax: 858-576-6564
Website: www.acefitness.org
E-mail: support@acefitness.org

American Heart Association (AHA)
7272 Greenville Ave.
Dallas, TX 75231
Toll-Free: 800-AHA-USA-1 (800-242-8721)
Phone: 214-570-5978
Fax: 214-706-1551
Website: www.heart.org

American Lung Association

55 W. Wacker Dr.
Ste. 1150
Chicago, IL 60601
Toll-Free: 800-LUNGUSA (800-548-8252)
Website: www.lung.org/about-us/contact-us.html
E-mail: info@lung.org

The American Medical Athletic Association (AMAA)

4405 E.W. Hwy
Ste. 405
Bethesda, MD 20814
Toll-Free: 800-776-2732
Phone: 301-913-9517
Fax: 301-913-9520
Website: www.amaasportsmed.org

The American Medical Society for Sports Medicine (AMSSM)

4000 W. 114th St.
Ste. 100
Leawood, KS 66211
Phone: 913-327-1415
Fax: 913-327-1491
Website: www.amssm.org

American Orthopaedic Foot & Ankle Society (AOFAS)

Orthopaedic Foot & Ankle Foundation
9400 W. Higgins Rd.
Ste. 220
Rosemont, IL 60018-4975
Toll-Free: 800-235-4855
Phone: 847-698-4654
Fax: 847-692-3315
Website: www.aofas.org/about/Pages/Contact-Us.aspx
E-mail: aofasinfo@aofas.org

American Orthopaedic Society for Sports Medicine (AOSSM)
9400 W. Higgins Rd.
Ste. 300
Rosemont, IL 60018
Toll-Free: 877-321-3500
Phone: 847-292-4900
Fax: 847-292-4905
Website: www.sportsmed.org

American Osteopathic Academy of Sports Medicine (AOASM)
2424 American Ln.
Madison, WI 53704
Phone: 608-443-2477
Fax: 608-443-2474
Website: www.aoasm.org/contact

American Physical Therapy Association (APTA)
1111 N. Fairfax St.
Alexandria, VA 22314-1488
Toll-Free: 800-999-APTA (800-999-2782)
Phone: 703-684-APTA (703-684-2782)
Fax: 703-684-7343
Website: www.apta.org/ContactUs
E-mail: learningcenter@apta.org

American Podiatric Medical Association (APMA)
9312 Old Georgetown Rd.
Bethesda, MD 20814-1621
Phone: 301-581-9200
Website: www.apma.org

American Running Association (ARA)
4405 E.W. Hwy
Ste. 405
Bethesda, MD 20814
Toll-Free: 800-776-2732
Fax: 301-913-9520
Website: www.americanrunning.org

American Society for Surgery of the Hand (ASSH)
822 W. Washington Blvd.
Chicago, IL 60607
Phone: 312-880-1900
Fax: 847-384-1435
Website: www.assh.org/About-ASSH/Contact-Us
E-mail: info@assh.org

Aquatic Exercise Association (AEA)
P.O. Box 1695
Brunswick, GA 31521-1695
Toll-Free: 888-232-9283
Phone: 941-486-8600
Fax: 941-486-8820
Website: www.aeawave.com/AboutUs/ContactAEA.aspx

Asthma and Allergy Foundation of America (AAFA)
8201 Corporate Dr.
Ste. 1000
Landover, MD 20785
Toll-Free: 800-7-ASTHMA (800-727-8462)
Website: www.aafa.org
E-mail: info@aafa.org

Cardiovascular Research Foundation (CRF)
1700 Bdwy.
Ninth Fl.
New York, NY 10019
Phone: 646-434-4500
Website: www.crf.org
E-mail: info@crf.org

Disabled Sports USA (DS/USA)
451 Hungerford Dr.
Ste. 608
Rockville, MD 20850
Phone: 301-217-0960
Fax: 301-217-0968
Website: www.disabledsportsusa.org/contact-us
E-mail: info@dsusa.org

Gatorade Sports Science Institute (GSSI)

617 W. Main St.
Barrington, IL 60010
Toll-Free: 800-616-GSSI (800-616-4774)
Website: www.gssiweb.com

HealthyWomen

P.O. Box 430
Red Bank, NJ 07701
Toll-Free: 877-986-9472
Phone: 732-530-3425
Fax: 732-865-7225
Website: www.healthywomen.org/about-us/contact-us
E-mail: info@healthywomen.org

IDEA Health & Fitness Association

10190 Telesis Ct.
San Diego, CA 92121
Toll-Free: 800-999-4332 ext. 7
Phone: 858-535-8979 ext. 7
Fax: 619-344-0380
Website: www.ideafit.com/contact
E-mail: contact@ideafit.com

International Fitness Association (IFA)

12472 Lake Underhill Rd.
Ste. 341
Orlando, FL 32828
Toll-Free: 800-227-1976
Phone: 407-579-8610
Website: www.ifafitness.com

National Alliance for Youth Sports (NAYS)

2050 Vista Pkwy
West Palm Beach, FL 33411
Toll-Free: 800-688-KIDS (800-688-5437)
Fax: 561-684-2546
Website: www.nays.org/about/about-nays/contact-us
E-mail: nays@nays.org

National Association for Health and Fitness (NAHF)

10 Kings Mill Ct.
Albany, NY 12205-3632
Phone: 518-456-1058
Website: www.physicalfitness.org/contact-us.html
E-mail: aerobic2@aol.com

National Athletic Trainers' Association (NATA)

1620 Valwood Pkwy
Ste. 115
Carrollton, TX 75006
Toll-Free: 800-879-6282
Phone: 214-637-6282
Fax: 214-637-2206
Website: www.nata.org/contact

National Center for Sports Safety (NCSS)

2316 First Ave. S.
Birmingham, AL 35233
Toll-Free: 866-508-NCSS (866-508-6277)
Phone: 205-329-7535
Website: www.sportssafety.org/contact
E-mail: info@sportssafety.org

National Center on Physical Activity and Disability (NCHPAD)

4000 Ridgeway Dr.
Birmingham, AL 35209
Toll-Free: 800-900-8086
Fax: 205-313-7475
Website: www.nchpad.org/Contactus
E-mail: email@nchpad.org

National Coalition for Promoting Physical Activity (NCPPA)

1150 Connecticut Ave. N.W.
Ste. 300
Washington, DC 20036
Phone: 202-454-7521
Website: www.ncppa.org/about-us?qt-about_us=2#qt-about_us
E-mail: ayanna@ncppa.org

National Osteoporosis Foundation (NOF)
1150 17th St. N.W., Ste. 850
Washington, DC 20036
Toll-Free: 800-231-4222
Phone: 202-223-2226
Fax: 202-223-2237
Website: www.nof.org/privacy-policy
E-mail: info@nof.org

National Strength and Conditioning Association (NSCA)
1885 Bob Johnson Dr.
Colorado Springs, CO 80906
Toll-Free: 800-815-6826
Phone: 719-632-6722
Fax: 719-632-6367
Website: www.nsca.com/contact-us
E-mail: nsca@nsca.com

North American Spine Society (NASS)
7075 Veterans Blvd.
Burr Ridge, IL 60527
Toll-Free: 866-960-6277
Phone: 630-230-3600
Fax: 630-230-3700
Website: www.spine.org/WhoWeAre/ContactUs.aspx

PE Central
2516 Blossom Trl W.
Blacksburg, VA 24060
Phone: 678-764-2536
Fax: 866-776-9170
Website: www.pecentral.org/contactus.html
E-mail: pec@pecentral.org

Prevent Sports Eye Injuries
211 W. Wacker Dr.
Ste. 1700
Chicago, IL 60606
Toll-Free: 800-331-2020
Website: www.preventblindness.org/contact-us
E-mail: info@preventblindness.org

Society of Health and Physical Educators (SHAPE America)
1900 Association Dr.
Reston, VA 20191
Toll-Free: 800-213-7193
Phone: 703-476-3400
Fax: 703-476-9527
Website: www.shapeamerica.org/about/contactus.cfm

University of Pittsburgh Medical Center (UPMC) Sports Medicine
200 Lothrop St.
Pittsburgh, PA 15213-2582
Toll-Free: 800-533-UPMC (800-533-8762)
Phone: 412-647-UPMC (412-647-8762)
Website: www.upmc.com/contact/Pages/default.aspx

Women's Sports Foundation
Eisenhower Park 1899 Hempstead Tpke
Ste. 400
East Meadow, NY 11554
Toll-Free: 800-227-3988
Phone: 516-542-4700
Fax: 516-542-0095
Website: www.womenssportsfoundation.org/privacy-policy
E-mail: info@WomensSportsFoundation.org

Chapter 64

Resources For More Information About Specific Sports And Activities

Amateur Athletic Union Basketball

P.O. Box 22409
Lake Buena Vista, FL 32830
Toll-Free: 800-AAU-4USA (800-228-4872)
Phone: 407-934-7200
Fax: 407-934-7242
Website: www.aausports.org/basketball

American Hiking Society (AHS)

8605 Second Ave.
Silver Spring, MD 20910
Toll-Free: 800-972-8608
Phone: 301-565-6704
Fax: 301-565-6704
Website: www.americanhiking.org/contact-us
E-mail: Info@AmericanHiking.org

About This Chapter: Resources in this chapter were compiled from several sources deemed reliable; all contact information was verified and updated in September 2017.

American Running Association (ARA)

4405 E.W. Hwy
Ste. 405
Bethesda, MD 20814
Toll-Free: 800-776-2732 (ext. 13 or 12)
Fax: 301-913-9520
Website: www.americanrunning.org/m/contact

American Whitewater (AW)

P.O. Box 1540
Cullowhee, NC 28723
Toll-Free: 866-262-8429
Phone: 828-586-1930
Fax: 828-586-2840
Website: www.americanwhitewater.org/content/Wiki/aw:contact_us
E-mail: info@americanwhitewater.org

American Youth Soccer Organization (AYSO)

19750 S. Vermont Ave.
Ste. 200
Torrance, CA 90502
Toll-Free: 800-USA-AYSO (800-872-2976)
Fax: 310-525-1155
Website: www.ayso.org/aboutayso/contact.htm#.Wbjx4t8xDrc

Aquatic Exercise Association (AEA)

P.O. Box 1695
Brunswick, GA 31521-1695
Toll-Free: 888-232-9283
Phone: 941-486-8600
Fax: 941-486-8820
Website: www.aeawave.com/AboutUs/ContactAEA.aspx

College and Junior Tennis

Port Washington Tennis Academy
100 Harbor Rd.
Port Washington, NY 11050
Phone: 516-883-6601
Fax: 516-883-5241
Website: www.collegeandjuniortennis.com/contact.htm
E-mail: info@collegeandjuniortennis.com

Dance/USA

1029 Vermont Ave. N.W.
Ste. 400
Washington, DC 20005
Phone: 202-833-1717
Fax: 202-833-2686
Website: www.danceusa.org

Inline Skating Resource Center

Website: www.iisa.org
E-mail: contact@iisa.org

International Skateboarding Federation (ISF)

P.O. Box 57
Woodward, PA 16882
Phone: 814-883-5635
Fax: 814-349-5413
Website: www.international skateboardingfederation.org

Little League® Baseball and Softball

539 U.S. Route 15 Hwy
P.O. Box 3485
Williamsport, PA 17701-0485
Phone: 570-326-1921
Fax: 570-326-1074
Website: www.littleleague.org/learn/about/contacts.htm

National Scholastic Surfing Association (NSSA)

P.O. Box 495
Huntington Beach, CA 92648
Phone: 714-906-7423
Website: www.nssa.org/newsmanager/templates/NSSAArticleShort.
aspx?articleid=34&zoneid=9

NFL Rush Safety & Privacy

Attn: NFL Legal Department
345 Park Ave.
New York, NY 10154
Phone: 212-450-2000
Website: www.nflrush.com/privacy/?icampaign=nflrush-main_nav_bar-global-about
E-mail: nflrushprivacy@nfl.com

Surfrider Foundation

P.O. Box 6010
San Clemente, CA 92674-6010
Phone: 949-492-8170
Fax: 949-492-8142
Website: www.surfrider.org/pages/contact-us
E-mail: info@surfrider.org

U.S. Figure Skating Association (USFSA)

20 First St.
Colorado Springs, CO 80906
Phone: 719-635-5200
Fax: 719-635-9548
Website: www.usfsa.org
E-mail: info@usfigureskating.org

U.S. Kids Golf

3040 Northwoods Pkwy
Norcross, GA 30071
Toll-Free: 888-3-US KIDS (888-387-5437)
Phone: 770-441-3077
Fax: 770-448-3069
Website: www.uskidsgolf.com/contact
E-mail: customerservice@uskidsgolf.com

U.S. Ski and Snowboard Association (USSA)

1 Victory Ln.
P.O. Box 100
Park City, UT 84060
Phone: 435-649-9090
Fax: 435-649-3613
Website: www.ussa.org/contact

U.S. Youth Soccer

9220 World Cup Way
Frisco, TX 75033
Toll-Free: 800-4SOCCER (800-476-2237)
Phone: 972-334-9300
Fax: 972-334-9960
Website: www.usyouthsoccer.org

U.S. Youth Volleyball League (USYVL)

2771 Plaza Del Amo
Ste. 808
Torrance, CA 90503
Toll-Free: 888-988-7985
Phone: 310-212-7008
Fax: 310-212-7182
Website: www.usyvl.org/about-usyvl/contact-us
E-mail: info@usyvl.org

USA Baseball

1030 Swabia Ct.
Ste. 201
Durham, NC 27703
Phone: 919-474-8721
Website: www.usabaseball.com/about/staff
E-mail: info@usabaseball.com

USA Cycling

210 USA Cycling Pt.
Ste. 100
Colorado Springs, CO 80919
Phone: 719-434-4200
Website: www.usacycling.org/usa-cycling-staff-contacts-directory.htm
E-mail: help@usacycling.org

USA Diving

1060 N. Capitol Ave.
Ste. E-310
Indianapolis, IN 46204
Phone: 317-237-5252
Fax: 317-237-5257
Website: www.teamusa.org/usa-diving/about-us/contact-us

USA Gymnastics

130 E. Washington St.
Ste. 700
Indianapolis, IN 46204
Toll-Free: 800-345-4719
Phone: 317-237-5050
Fax: 317-237-5069
Website: www.usagym.org/pages/aboutus/pages/staffdirectory.html
E-mail: membership@usagym.org

USA Jump Rope

P.O. Box 569
Huntsville, TX 77342-0569
Phone: 936-295-3332
Fax: 936-295-3309
Website: www.usajumprope.org/page-22-contacts.html
E-mail: info@usajumprope.org

USA Softball

USA Softball Hall of Fame Stadium Complex
2801 N.E. 50th St.
Oklahoma City, OK 73111
Phone: 405-424-5266
Website: www.teamusa.org/usa-softball/about/contact-us

USA Swimming

1 Olympic Plaza
Colorado Springs, CO 80909
Phone: 719-866-4578
Website: www.usaswimming.org/Home/about/usa-swimming
E-mail: info@usaswimming.org

USA Water Ski

1251 Holy Cow Rd.
Polk City, FL 33868-8200
Phone: 863-324-4341
Fax: 863-325-8259
Website: www.usawaterski.org
E-mail: memberservices@usawaterski.org

Index

Index

Page numbers that appear in *Italics* refer to tables or illustrations. Page numbers that have a small 'n' after the page number refer to citation information shown as Notes. Page numbers that appear in **Bold** refer to information contained in boxes within the chapters.

A

H

I

Y